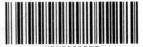
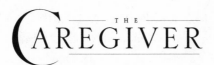

THE
CAREGIVER

6-24-09

T H E
CAREGIVER

A LIFE WITH ALZHEIMER'S
AARON ALTERRA

Foreword by ARTHUR KLEINMAN

ILR Press
AN IMPRINT OF
CORNELL UNIVERSITY PRESS
ITHACA AND LONDON

First published in cloth and paperback, Steerforth Press, 1999
First printing, Cornell Paperbacks, 2007

Printed in the United States of America

Library of Congress Cataloging-in-Publication Data
Alterra, Aaron.
    The Caregiver : a life with Alzheimer's / Aaron Alterra.
        p. cm. — (The culture and politics of health care work) (Cornell
paperbacks)
    Originally published : South Royalton, Vt. : Steerforth Press, 1999.
    ISBN 978-0-8014-7434-7 (pbk. : alk. paper)
    1. Alzheimer's disease—Patients—Care. 2. Caregivers. I. Title.
II. Series. III. Series: Cornell paperbacks.
    RC523.A365 2007
    616.8'31—dc22   2007033207

Author's note: Everything in this book is true, but it is all so close
to me that I would not have been able to write it without changing
names and certain identifiable circumstances and by taking cover
under the pen name Aaron Alterra.—E. S. Goldman

Cornell University Press strives to use environmentally
responsible suppliers and materials to the fullest extent possible
in the publishing of its books. Such materials include vegetable-
based, low-VOC inks and acid-free papers that are recycled,
totally chlorine-free, or partly composed of nonwood fibers. For
further information, visit our website at
www.cornellpress.cornell.edu.

Paperback printing   10 9 8 7 6 5 4 3 2 1

For Virginia

CONTENTS

The Caregiver is that perfect small book, the one that tells a difficult, deeply human story, simply, beautifully, without wasted words or embellished affect. The writing is so direct, so pure, that the story steps out of the pages and enters into the reader's senses like an immediate experience of the existential. You carry that experience with you as if it were yours, not the writer's. You know it will remain iconic. When you think of Alzheimer's you will reexperience, reimagine this story.

Here is a writer's sensibility of caregiving for a spouse: a husband nursing a wife. (Research tells us this often goes less well than when a wife nurses a husband.) The early days of uncertainty and denial before a diagnosis tolls the dangers ahead;

the slow but inevitable unmaking of cognition and personhood and remaking of relationships; the transition from unbearable catastrophe to all-too-bearable disability; the transfiguring of personal tragedy into collective bereavement for our common humanity; all things real and important that matter more than hope are found in these pages.

"It plays on a different reed," says the author's spouse, fighting through dementia to find a startlingly original expression for her disorder's unique emotions, which join together through Alzheimer's toward shared human ends.

The dawning recognition today is that there is no typical case of Alzheimer's disease. The over 5 million Americans with this neurodegeneration experience the illness differently. Trajectories vary so greatly and proceed at such greatly individual paces that the natural course of the brain degeneration is as personal as an autobiography and as social as the local worlds where families and facilities create distinctive histories. It is only recently that people with Alzheimer's have found voices to object to being silenced, treated as if they were not there, made invisible. Caregivers—we are talking of tens of millions for Alzheimer's and other neurodegenerative disorders—are understood to bear a huge burden of suffering. Their stories have become emblematic of the crucial recognition that Alzheimer's is transpersonal. The locus of suffering is somewhere between the patient and the caregiver.

The English writer John Bayley's *Elegy for Iris* recounts Iris Murdoch's experience of dementia and Bayley's unflagging commitment to nurse his extraordinary wife until the end. An arresting book, its heroine is such a larger-than-life figure that the reader just knows this is not a tale of the ordinary. *The Caregiver*'s protagonist, in contrast, is an ordinary woman, closer to the reader's world.

One of this book's most poignant insights is that the critical knowledge of the illness experience does not reside in the medical profession. Expert knowledge of Alzheimer's belongs to spouses, children, friends, and the professional companions, aides, and nurses who do the actual caregiving—meaning, everything from driving, walking with, reading to, feeding, bathing, and just being there for people whose brain is no longer capable of letting them be independent. *The Caregiver* discloses the powerful truth that Alzheimer's does not create a uniform set of losses. Some cognitive, sensory, and motor functions are lost, but others are changed, some are spared, and some are even enhanced or gained anew. The living and the caregiving are all about going through these changes on a daily basis and over the long term.

I am myself a caregiver. My wife's neurodegenerative disorder seems to combine elements of Alzheimer's disease with others that more closely resemble those that Oliver Sacks described in the case of the man who mistook his wife for a hat. I recognize myself in so much of what the author of *The Caregiver* has written that I can attest to its authenticity and its wisdom.

Emmanuel Levinas—the influential French theologian and ethicist—insists that the ethical must always precede the epistemological or ontological in human relationships. How we know and what our being is about take second place to the affirmation of the other and responses to the other's suffering. And that suffering only takes on its ethical significance as we face it, engage it, and make it over into our reality, our lives. Caregiving is at the core of what it means to be human. The caregiver is you and me, all of us. Read this book, because it not only illuminates caregiving; it clarifies why caregiving matters so greatly for Alzheimer's disease and for all the other health catastrophes that transfigure our lives. Caregiving is what we are here for; we are all caregivers. What makes this book exceptional is that it is written by that rare caregiver who has managed to work through and fully understand what is happening to him and who tells his story so illuminatingly that we are enabled to draw the deepest lessons for living.

ARTHUR KLEINMAN
Professor of Medical Anthropology and Psychiatry,
Harvard University
Author of *What Really Matters: Living A Moral Life amidst Uncertainty and Danger*

THE CAREGIVER

1

Forgetting How Things Are Done

CONSIDERING HOW SECOND-class my own memory is, I was slow to be concerned about Stella's. We had been married a week when I drove the car out of the garage and got halfway to town before realizing that Stella was waiting in front of the house for me to pick her up. That was sixty years ago. Wives don't readily give up such advantageous stories.

My handicap had not been recently acquired. I couldn't re-member parts in high-school plays, or ever carry a punch line longer than a few days. Invincibly confident that the mo-mentum of telling will force the point into my mouth the way the ends of stories materialize as I type, I have come up empty before audiences and asked if anybody in the house knows what I'm supposed to say next. When I reread today what I wrote only a year or two ago, I am surprised by the turns sen-tences take; it is as if I had never before seen them; it was not much different when I was younger.

Bringing myself into the story this way is only to offer a fairly convincing reason why I did not take Stella's memory lapses very seriously. Not having been looking for anything like that, I can't say exactly when it began for her.

I noticed indecisiveness, as if she had made up her mind enough times in all these years about how many spoons of coffee to brew, what kind of vase to put flowers in, and did not want to think very much about it anymore. She opened drawers and closed them without apparent purpose. Minor hesitations occurred in her driving decisions: which lane? what gear? why am I on this road going in this direction? The kitchen is a gallery of opportunities to forget salt, butter, onions in familiar recipes. A film of preoccupation occasionally settled on her. When I tried to penetrate it without putting on a show of clinical concern, she said she felt fine. She changed to more alphabetical vitamins.

It did not seem to me significant that at an advanced age Stella forgot the Spanish word for ———, the name of that woman who ———, the title of the book about ———. Months passed while I adjusted to no longer relying on her for the titles of books, the names of places we had visited, the names of people we didn't see very often. Before there was a recognizable sign of anything except that she was eighty years old I realized I could no longer rely on my wife to repair my memory, and that she had begun to bring me the kinds of questions I had always brought to her.

"You're changing the rules," I said amiably. "I'm supposed to ask *you* the names of people we met once."

"Well, I'm asking," she said, not as amiably as I.

"It shouldn't bother you to forget the name of somebody you met once. At our age you're allowed."

It wasn't only the loss of a casual acquaintance's name that bothered her. She had also, for a long second, blanked the name of her oldest grandchild. She was in no hurry to circulate that information in the family.

It isn't easy to convince people that you are losing an extraordinary amount of memory, especially if at the same time you want to keep it to yourself. You may not be able to tell the extraordinary from the ordinary. They think you exaggerate. They don't hear you. They want to talk you out of it.

Mention to your daughter who is half your age that you now forget a few things and she immediately tells you that she forgets: words won't come off the tip of her tongue; she writes a lot of notes to herself these days. Modest claims of forgetfulness are tokens of intergenerational solidarity.

When we get older we forget a little more. It's on the curve. Before Alzheimer's — notoriously a disease of lost memory — is pseudo-Alz, which is simply lost memory. I saw my part as minimizing any anxieties she might have. I had lived with a similar problem.

There may never have been a beginning. The thing itself may have been there always, moving subterraneously along the nerves, choosing hesitantly, forgetting, before acknowledging its medical name. Each hesitant choice, each forgetfulness may have been early advice of more profound disability to come. Termites show only a few dead wings on a porch step, a flight on a spring day you may not be home to see, while substance is being hollowed to dry tissue. Then a corner post gives way and a wall sags.

That it is in the genes, evading notice, was for a while thought to account for most cases. The particular fact the diagnosing doctor wanted to know was, Was something like this — not necessarily named this, but this kind of behavior — evident in a parent, a grandparent, an aunt, or an uncle? Did they lose their memories? Did they become helpless in their old age? Did a relative take care of them? Did they go to nursing homes, whatever such institutions were then called? No, Stella said to all that. The questions are still asked in diagnostic interviews but the prevailing opinion has become that not more than one or two cases in ten begin in faulty genes. Authorities speak now of diet, environment, infection, habit, lifestyle.

As I had always taken my forgetfulness as a fact of nature, like my shoe size, and had attributed accelerating losses to old age, I took her condition to be comparable, at most a frustration, not a disease. It was one of those things . . . Don't worry about it . . . Join the club.

If you have some years on you, as I do, you have been in a familiar place and stopped on dead center for a long moment and muttered, Where am I going? Why am I in this mall? Which is the save key? The other morning I enjoyed a remarkably smooth shave and in my mind reconstructed the sequence of showering and soaping before it came to me that the blade cover was still on the razor. Nothing is as good as a layer of plastic between razor and beard to make the perfect shave imagined by advertising copywriters. Can such anecdotes be what we are talking about when we ask, When did you first notice it? Is the same thing working in me at eighty-five that emerged to catch Stella at eighty, and if it is, will I outrun it to the more lucid and ordinary end of heart failure or cancer?

It is not merely a matter of curiosity. The earlier the treatment, the more equal the contest between disease and drug. The available drugs do not cure. They may delay. The best possible years may be prolonged.

"True," said Loughrand, Stella's physician. "But, the earlier the symptoms the more likely are the available physicians to shrug them off."

Stella's brain soon retrieved the name of her grandchild. I imagined a brain of infinite pathways ingeniously disposed to make the necessary detours around disruptions. Perhaps the passage of information would be slower, as walking becomes slower with age, but adjustments would be made and the brain would get where it intended to go. My first perception of what I was there to do — before what possessed Stella was given a name and before I became her caregiver — was to replace her lost words from my remaining supply: *basil... zinnias... Penang... Puvis de Chavannes.* Oddly, her losses seemed always to be nouns, the names of things, people, places.

I say "oddly" because the words lost in my head were not only nouns but also the more subtle parts of speech. I tried to account for our not asking each other for verbs and adjectives and it came to this: she was a music person and I was a word person. Typically, she wrote letters. Letters do not need an extraordinary supply of modifying words. She was a consumer of nouns colored with a minimum of familiar verbs. I thanked her when she spared some nouns for me, and rifled dictionaries and thesauruses and looked out windows for the rest.

When Stella first became conscious that she was losing words, I did not want her to think she was falling behind.

Words were only words. Behind them was intact intelligence. Prefacing the suggestion with disclaimers — neither of us is as young as we used to be; I forget even more than you do — I counseled her to slow down when her memory slowed, expect less of herself. I did more of the chores husbands are invited to assume. I sliced bread. I made salads. I microwaved soup. We began to eat out more often.

Still, I would say she was living a normal life in a normal way with a little less intensity; giving a little more thought before putting one foot in front of the other, but within a range of the normal, the expected.

In her company for the first time, you would identify a reserved, competent, elderly woman, one who chose her clothes well, whose walking was somewhat infirm. Those who knew her better saw the edges of what I saw: Stella really needed an arm these days to get her across the restaurant floor, to get her down and settled in her chair and then back up again. A little patience was needed to stay with her as she looked for a word or veered from the point. After all, she was eighty.

One incident became a milestone for me, a day I counted from. She looked into my office and asked if I would like turnips for dinner. I knew that meant turnips from Nickerson's farm, a few miles down the road, the sweetest turnips in the world. The dinner that came to the table was one boiled turnip. Furtively I established that nothing had been forgotten on top of the range or in the oven. Nothing in the refrigerator looked like it had been intended to come out.

She is preoccupied, I assured myself. She had been invited to do the centerpiece performance at the forthcoming Festival of the Arts and was calling her cellist friends around the state to perform with her the Bachianas Brasileiro that Villa-Lobos wrote for eight cellos. She had often spoken of the piece with high artistic appetite but never had a chance to play it. "Eight cellos!" she exclaimed gleefully, eyes snapping, her strong cellist hands shaping it in her imagination. She ordered the music, began marking parts. Lost words were nothing compared to found music.

I ceded the priority of eight cellos over a more comprehensive plan for dinner, but I remembered how unremarkable it seemed to Stella that a turnip was all anyone should expect.

What else? Usually I drove when we were out together. Occasionally she dropped me at the library or the dentist's or I left my car for a job at the garage, and when she picked me up in her car it was convenient for me to get into the passenger's seat. It seemed to me that for fleeting instants her driving skills lapsed. She was unsure of the sequence of getting the car in motion: key, pedal, lights, wipers, gear, gas. She was momentarily uncertain about which road to take, which lane to be in for the turn. A street is a noun. Getting home is modifiers and verbs. In a lazy way I rehearsed emergencies, kicking her foot off the gas pedal, reaching for the wheel, grabbing the handbrake. Her flutters of indecision passed as the normal rhythms of driving took over, passed quickly, and came again.

She surged the gas. The car didn't move.

"You're in neutral."

"I know how to drive a car."

I didn't say, "Nevertheless you're in neutral." The way things had begun to go between us, her next line would have been, "Please get off my back" or a counter-accusation, "Last week you went through a red light." My part would be that as to the first I was trying to be helpful, and as to the second it was not up to wives to agree with traffic cops in close cases. The light had been yellow when I got into the intersection.

Anyhow, that was last week and I didn't claim to be perfect. Right now the car was in neutral.

Our dispositions had always been to stay on the same page, have it out on the page, and turn the page together. I was adjusting to a Stella who flailed out defensively even when she must have known she was wrong. I had prepared for something like this during her menopause, but Stella had made that transition rather easily. As no marriage is served by establishing who is right and who is wrong no matter what, I bit my tongue and gave it time.

But I began to grasp that dwelling on loss of vocabulary had misled me. To be more exact, what was happening was a loss of the sense of how things were connected, where she was in the flow. In a metaphorical sense, the nouns of her life remained — *brake* and *gas pedal* were there; *turnip* was there, *dinner* was there; but other parts of speech — connections and nuances to bind them into meaningful processes — were relaxing. I looked inside myself and could not find anything like that.

At four o'clock one afternoon she looked into my workroom and said dinner was ready. Dinner at four in the afternoon? Maybe for farmers. Maybe for people in Iowa. I was still working. Maybe she had misread the time. She was standing beside me. I looked at her wristwatch. Four. I showed her my desk clock. Four. She was unimpressed. Dinner was ready. I pointed out the window to the light that hung on in the January afternoon. The sky was white, the colors of roofs and fields could be made out. At our usual dinner hour neighborly window lights would break the darkness. This was not very interesting to her. Dinner was ready.

Attached to the kitchen range is a clock that adjusts its hour and minute hands to a random new time whenever the oven timer is set, unless the setting is done with a safecracker's sensitive fingers. The clock can never be relied on to tell the true time. (The clock's designer has a partner who put the horn on the perimeter of the steering wheel so that in an emergency it has to be chased like a wild squirrel. Another partner imprints important instructions on the plastic bodies of products where they are as unreadable as braille to the sighted.) I walked back to the kitchen with her. The clock happened to be right. Four o'clock. Stella saw nothing irregular about dinner at four and was irritated when I asked her to cover my plate, I would microwave it later. I was working.

The tag "short-term memory loss" as the characteristic Alzheimer's symptom also misled me. The phrase has an inherent bias toward recent events — yesterday, last month, year-before-last. It didn't hint at an early loss of faculties that have been exercised since childhood. The names of girls she had gone to school with, the names of herbs that had been in her father's garden were not recently acquired memories. What could be longer term for Stella, who had been raised in a traditional home, than knowing how to cook? When had she learned to drive a car? In Pennsylvania we were licensed at sixteen.

Today there are books, articles, television and radio programs, many ways for a layman to be enlightened about the disease. The Alzheimer's Association has chapters in more than two hundred central, staffed locations with counsel and racks of literature for the asking; there are more than ten times that many active caregiver groups whose meeting places are known in town halls and in local senior centers.

I know now that a few Alzheimer's articles had been in the papers then too, and when I look at copyright dates I see that there were books, but I had read nothing that described the connection between short-term memory loss and images of vacant senility that I could in any way relate to Stella.

The better-known explanation of her symptoms was that she had suffered a small stroke. Nineteen ninety-four was the year of news stories about the incidence, the medications, the diets and science of stroke and its less jeopardizing twin, transient ischemic attack (TIA).

TIA provided a possible explanation for changes in Stella, and now that I had a word for it, the condition became more apparent. Instead of settling down at a level we could get used to, her decline was accelerating. Maybe she had had one or two of those quiet strokes. She would not think about things like that going on in herself. The only medical news Stella was alert to was about breast cancer. Her mother's last illness was cancer. Her older sister had had benign polyps removed.

TIA was something to see a doctor about. How to get Stella to see one without alarming her was on my mind when our son telephoned that he had a break in his schedule and was coming down for a day.

Our children live in different cities, raising their own children, but we are a close family and often visit in one direction or the other. We had all been together for Christmas. They had not noticed anything that couldn't be explained by their mother having passed her eightieth birthday. Her vagueness they translated to tiredness; she should get more rest. In the two months since then the episodes had become more frequent. What I told them on the phone was guarded. I intercepted Damon in the driveway and asked him to keep an eye on his mother and let me know if he saw anything that disturbed him.

"Like what?"

Well, she was getting a little rocky. She did not seem to be concentrating well. I had become used to the rhythm of her practice and she was breaking short, sitting and looking at a page of music for a long time.

Damon has an engineer's mind and education. "What's a long time?"

"Fifteen or twenty minutes. Not really reading it, just looking at it. She gets a little lost in the kitchen about how long things take to cook. She runs out of things like milk. She always had a good memory, but now it isn't as reliable as it was."

"Whose is? Mine isn't. Mom should write herself notes."

"You talk like your sister."

He is a dutiful and observant son. He and his mother love each other very much. I had said enough. Her demeanor and conversation were normal for ordinary society, but he would notice small changes in the way she moved; hesitations about direction, about what to do next, that would be unnoticed by a stranger. We were at the door and Stella took possession of him.

He saw the careful — programmed — way she let herself down into a chair and asked if her arthritis was acting up. When it did it settled around her repaired hip joints. "Oh not so bad." She told him what pill she took. I waited. Arthritis was not the subject. In the next few hours he would make other observations. He heard her lose the name of an old family friend. The subject was more than lost words.

They went to the store to buy fish for dinner. I excused myself to clean up my desk. Mother and son should be together without me there to absorb conversation. Stella hungered for time with her children. She might say things to him she didn't say to me. Damon and I would talk about it. He is acute. We would be on the same page. I realized too late I hadn't told him to let his mother drive.

When they come back Stella went to the bedroom to nap and Damon pulled a chair around on the porch so we could look at each other while we talked.

"I kept an eye on Mom. She isn't quite —" he needed a word, "all right, is she?"

"Nobody is *all* right at our age."

"She has some kind of memory problem."

I had gotten that far months ago. I wanted him to see more. "Doesn't everybody? I tried for an hour yesterday to think of the word for the two-bladed instrument that cuts paper."

"Ruler," he said. "I used to cut pages with a six-inch celluloid ruler I used as a bookmark. You never have to cut book pages anymore."

Bantering between us — he in his middle age, I in the decade after the biblical allotment — is as much a mark of the family as are his mother's black Spanish eyelashes and hazel eyes in the setting of pale skin and wheat hair. The family mark is on both children in those ways, and in the respectful manner of their rebellions, even in their marriages to the wrong girl and the wrong boy, which time — more than thirty married years now for both children! — showed to be the wisest possible choices, as the marriage from disapproving traditions proved itself for their parents.

"How do you know celluloid? I thought any plastic you remembered would be postnylon."

"Celluloid, Isinglass were words you and mother used."

"A ruler doesn't have two blades."

"Celluloid rulers are thin. You can cut with both edges."

You don't win many arguments with Damon. He never did as well on multiple-choice tests as he would have had he relaxed and accepted the questions as creations of simpleminded inquisitors. He wrestled for answers as if a subtle deity challenged him across the table. He brought tests home and demanded that I agree with him: Wasn't this question unanswerable? Wasn't one answer as good as another? Wasn't his answer *better* than theirs? I agreed, but look at it this way: the point was not for them to find out what he knew but for him to find out what *they* knew.

Our habit of conversation may be circular but not to evade a point. He said, "It seems to me different from just losing words." He was getting there. "Tell me what you saw."

"Getting out of the car Mom unbuckled her seat belt. She took off her sunglasses and exchanged them for her regular glasses and fussed to get the case into her pocketbook. Then she rebuckled as if she expected us to drive away instead of having just got back. She didn't quite get it when I told her we weren't going, we were coming."

I had seen such reversals. Stella stopping for some reason in a process, starting up again in reverse until she caught herself. Or didn't catch herself. Socks on; pause; socks off. Sitting down for dinner, unfolding napkin, refolding napkin, standing up, pushing chair back. Reversing again as if nothing had happened. Maybe nothing had happened for her. It happened for the observer. I had thought *absentminded;* not as young as she used to be; cover for her; don't let it bug her.

"That was just now. When we started out she directed me to the store where she wanted to buy fish. Next to the bank."

"Your mother never buys fish there. That's Old Central Market where she gets groceries. She buys fish two blocks farther on, at Peterson's."

"I found that out. She looked bewildered. 'They've changed things,' she said."

They. An impulse to see fault in the environment, not in herself, something recent in her. I put her car in the garage one night when I saw a squall coming over the hill. Backing it out the next morning, Stella nicked the sideview mirror against the door frame, knocking it out of alignment. "You parked too close to the wall," she said. I thought that was comic. A driver wasn't supposed to just get in and go. A driver was supposed to look around. I laughed. "Well, you did," she said.

Damon said, "When we finished at the fish store she left her pocketbook on the counter. I noticed when she was already through the door and went back to get it. We drove home and there was the business with the seat belt. Is Mom losing some memory?"

Leaving things behind: pocketbooks, hats, gloves. Headed in wrong directions. "You're a smart fella. Did what you see add up to common, ordinary loss of memory?"

Damon is indeed a smart fella. His degree is in engineering. He is the American president of a Swedish ship charterer. His job is to know who needs a carrier for oil or grain and who has one available. He has to know what calls to make, where to be on the spot to make the deal, anywhere from Boston to Galveston. He has to know prices, markets and ports, rates of exchange, schedules. He has to be fast and reliable so people will prefer to do business with him. He was a good son concerned about his mother. Now that his attention was focused it wouldn't take him long to see that clichés about octogenarian vocabulary and memory loss didn't cover this case.

He said, "It's more like not connecting here to there. Losing track of relationships."

"You got it!" I told him about her rinsing out an empty jelly jar and putting the jar full of rinse water in the refrigerator. I told him about the cutlery drawer. "Your mother puts spoons in the knife bin. She puts knives in the fork bin. She never used to do anything like that. Your mother was always the soul of order."

I told him about her coming out of the bookstore and turning left toward the bank instead of right toward the post office where I said I would wait for her. When she didn't come by I looked for her in the logical stores, the library, the park. Nobody I knew to ask had seen her. I stopped a cruiser and asked the officer to put a call out for her. A policeman found her parked on Holman's Meadow Road. She told him she was trying to get home. She would have had to go around the world to get home by way of Holman's Meadow. She would have to go around the universe to get home while parked.

She told the officer I wasn't where I had told her to pick me up. I had forgotten her and gone somewhere.

"You did once," Damon said. "Is Mom aware of all this?"

"Sometimes yes, sometimes no, and sometimes I don't know. She has a peculiar reaction. She has picked up a mechanism that keeps her from admitting she's wrong even when she must know it. She kind of closes down and won't discuss it. There were a half dozen knots in her shoelace this morning. I asked her 'How come?' She wouldn't take the question. Just looked blank. Absented herself. Wouldn't discuss."

"Why do you want to discuss? Untie the knots and forget it."

"I'm getting there. I'm not there yet but I'm getting there."

"Mom says you're becoming bossy."

"I know. She says it to me."

To extricate myself from contesting such charges I had a mantra, *I thought I was being helpful*. When I observed myself smelling saintly of forbearance, I told myself to come off the high. Anyhow, our horizons of displeasure never extended more than a few hours. We heard early in our marriage about never going to sleep mad, tried it, and never broke the habit.

Damon said, "She says you tell her how to cook."

What was really happening was that she wanted me to help in the kitchen but on her terms, and I kept overrunning her pace. We have a tight galley kitchen. I reached across her, I went around. She didn't slice a carrot the way she used to, rattling from end to end like a chef. She cut a slice, repositioned the carrot, cut another slice, looked out the window, forgot she had been slicing a carrot, and began to brew the coffee. She took butter out of the refrigerator, closed the refrigerator, opened it again to put the butter back.

I spoke my mantra to Damon. "I try to be helpful. She can be two hours getting a meal together. I try to be subtle and maneuver her —"

He didn't like his father maneuvering his mother. It was not his image of their relationship. He had not been comfortable with the idea of his mother breaking down and was quick to scramble to other ground. "Mom appreciates that you're trying to help her, but maybe you ought to back off a little. It comes across to her as a power trip. Wouldn't it be a good idea to let her find her own pace?"

"It sounds easy. I'm not complaining. I'm just telling you what goes on."

"If you could work alongside her and just be meek?" He grinned at the absurdity. His image of his father was not meek. "And helpful?"

The subject had changed from his mother's condition to my role. I could not protest a son's chivalric emotion on his mother's behalf.

"You do the meek and helpful," I suggested. "Make the salad. Don't lift a finger to do anything else. See what goes on."

We came here a quarter century ago, hardly expecting these extra years. We had lived in big cities, worked where we needed others as they needed us. This is a country cottage made over for a woman with a cello, a man with a writing machine, and space for visiting family and friends. Dayrooms without interior walls surround the stone fireplace. The kitchen begins at the breakfast counter, the den at the back-to-back bookcases. Where walls have come out, skinned timbers carry the upper floor. Windows bring in bird feeders on somewhat squirrelproof poles, fallow early-winter gardens, thick nesting places in hemlock, box, rhododendron, heaths, heathers. Stella is besieged on this ground she chose.

I set the table while Damon found in the vegetable drawer what he wanted for a salad and Stella moved serenely from task to task with no methodical agenda. That she was now bent and finely wrinkled hardly diminished my satisfaction that her beauty had always been appropriate to the time of her life. Far from "the uneventful Cliveden profile" — V. S. Pritchett's phrase — a young suitor had expected to go with narrow shoulders and a face so close to the bone, Stella's hips were sudden, knuckled. A young therapist admired them last year: "Some hips!" From somebody in her business it was a serious compliment.

(If you are uncomfortable with the implication of the erotic attraction of a woman at eighty — eighty-five as I write this — suffer more: the sagging breasts, iconic of the destiny of an aged woman, draw the surface of globes taut so that in the midst of physical degradation the breast is as smooth as a bride's. I did not abdicate the nightly privilege of helping her undress until a year or so ago, in her fourth year of Alz, when an aide took over. I stand by. Stella no longer becomes entangled in a gown, her head in the sleeve, and calls, "Can you help me dear?" She accepts that garments are slipped off with only her passive participation. Still, when her head emerges through the neckline, she is in a game and, seeing me, grins to acknowledge that I am in it too.)

Damon and I talked about grandchildren and Damon's trip to Sweden and the cello concert. When she spoke Stella stopped what she was doing as if only one process at a time could get through and daydreamed before starting up again.

She looked through cookbooks and card files to find her recipe for baked fish, which even I knew. Put it in the glass baking dish. Put on some dabs of butter, salt and pepper, and a dusting of dried herbs from the second shelf down. Pour in some milk. She set the bake dial but not the temperature. The oven won't flame unless both dials are set. I asked if she wanted me to set the temperature. Stella said yes, not as if she had forgotten but as if it was the exact moment and she had been about to do it. When the timer bell rang for the fish she put a pot of water on to boil for rice. She took a box of frozen peas from the freezer. Preparing dinner was becoming a serial event.

"Why bother with that, Stell? Isn't the salad enough?"

We left her puttering in the kitchen and went to the television for the Michigan game, my school, but had barely settled in when I heard a slight exclamation and jumped toward what sounded like trouble. Stella was dabbing paper towels on the counter. A film of water spread slowly, wouldn't mop up as I expected a spill would, kept coming like an exudation of the vinyl surface, pooling and running over the metal edge, drooling to the floor. The mop towels were stained tan. The red light showed on the coffeemaker but there was no pot on the hot plate. I had to go through those instantaneous observations before my brain said Coffee! "Hey!" I exclaimed at the same time Damon yanked the cord from the wall socket. Stella had forgot to put the pot under the drip. She was not upset; bemused, rather, and, I think, taking into her memory that I had shouted.

We sat down for the TV news after dinner. I handed Stella the remote. We had had a new television set for several months. The state-of-the-art controls seemed to be unnecessarily cumbersome, but they were the product of the combined resources of two Fortune 500 companies and were what they were. The twenty-page manual was mostly concerned about how to save programs that came on when we weren't there. The many attractive possibilities of this function would have been too esoteric for Stella in her best year, and I had not been able to convey to her my hard-won knowledge of how to turn the thing on and off, how to change stations and volume and reach the blessed plateau of mute.

Damon took a sheet of paper from the stack at the computer and made a chart with bold lettering and arrows pointing to buttons. He is an engineer. I mumbled that I too had made charts, but his was doubtless better.

It was time for him to go. I walked him to his car.

"Don't you think Mom ought to see a doctor?"

"I'm tooling up to get it done. I don't want to alarm her."

Proposing to Stella that she see a doctor because of something as ordinary as *lost words,* as vague as *memory lapse,* even though she herself knew something was wrong, seemed to me to be anxiety-creating. Her back would go up. *"See a doctor about what?"*

We had no sense of present danger. Damon was as disturbed as I but there was no blood, no blemish, no lump, no searing pain, no pain at all, no midnight ride in an ambulance as there would be in our experience of urgency. In the telling the symptoms seem to have been all of Stella's life, but they were then only episodes in otherwise ordinary days. "Keep in touch," he said and put a comradely arm on my shoulder.

The next evening Marion was on the phone from Washington. Stella took the call. Like her brother, Marion is loving, dutiful, observant. She runs a social agency. She had to be in Boston for a meeting next week. She would be with us for a couple of days.

"That's wonderful," Stella said.

They talked until Marion asked to speak to me.

"What's going on, Dad?"

"You've been talking to your brother," I said.

"Of course. Can you and I talk?"

"We're always glad to see you. But, you know, I hope you aren't taking this trip especially to see us."

Stella made a face. It didn't bother her if her children had to come in from the moon. She didn't see them that often.

"You can't talk? Let's try. Wouldn't it be a good idea for you and Mother to sit down with somebody who is good on interpersonal relations? You must have somebody up there. If you don't know anybody, I could find a lead for you."

She saw it as a problem between her parents. A counselor knew the ropes. Counselors had degrees, they asked pertinent questions, made suggestions, mediated.

Stella and I had always backed away from such encounters. We were self-service psychologists. We had not needed counselors to get our children through the nineteen sixties and we certainly didn't need them for ourselves in our full maturity. We granted that many people lacked knowledge, resources, perspectives, and confidence; they needed third parties to help them through crises of parenting, marriage, menopause, and unemployment. We were not those people. People came to us for somebody to talk things through with. We sent checks to counseling agencies as we sent checks to the United Fund, as a duty of citizenship.

"Of course," I said.

Marion was surprised by the immediate affirmative. She knew her parents as the kind of people who did not go to counselors. We went to doctors. She had expected a longer argument.

"You'll do it?"

I had meant, Of course she would think counseling was a good idea. She was a social worker. I couldn't say it because Stella would hear *counseling* and ask what that was all about. I said, "We'll see."

She heard in my voice that I wasn't going to do it. "Oh Dad! Think about it. Will you call me at the office tomorrow morning when we can talk?"

"Sure. Basically, we're okay here."

"I know. I'll be there Thursday. Jerry wants to talk to you."

Talking to my son-in-law is a change of weather from talking to my daughter. She is ebullient, forward, giving; she goes to the net. Jerry stands in the backcourt and keeps hitting it back; he expects there will be an opening soon enough. He is an architect and also a paramedic on the rescue squad in his town. Reverse the priority: he is a paramedic and also an architect. Every tenth night he sleeps at the firehouse. If he were not fifty-some years old he might keep on taking courses and end as an M.D.

"What's going on with Stella?" His own mother was already Mom when he met Marion's parents. "Mrs." is stiff. Stella's rank in the hierarchy is implicit. "Can you talk?"

Stella had no more stake in the conversation and had left the room. Marion could pick us up on the other phone if she wanted to. "What can I say. Stell is getting older. She is a little rocky." I was getting used to saying phrases with *rocky* in them. It was noncommittal and inclusive, suggestive without being alarming. I could see him long distance, attentive, organized to listen. I heard him tool up to make me more forthcoming. I heard Marion click back on. "Is it forgetfulness? Is she missing appointments? Is it her walking?"

"Some of all that. She is not walking with much vigor, but she still does a half mile on the treadmill. She seems to find the surface reassuring. When she begs off the treadmill it's usually because her hips are getting painful. She went for a checkup to the orthopedist who did her hip replacements. Everything looks all right to him. He said not to be concerned about mild pain. Take a couple of aspirin. In certain weather arthritis may tend to gravitate toward the hip replacements. Keep exercising."

"Did he watch her walk?"

"Up and down the hall."

"Did she walk for him the way you noticed as a change?"

"Yes. Slowly and a little unsteadily. As if she wanted to be sure one foot was down before she moved the other one."

Jerry processed my answer. "He didn't say anything about that? Did he say she should see your family doctor?"

Marion said, "Did he recommend a neurologist?"

"No, he said the hip replacements were in good shape."

"They all read from their own book," Jerry said. "What else makes you say 'rocky'? We all forget things."

"I understand that. I'm not a hypochondriac. She has some memory problems, but I mean things like losing track of what she's doing in the kitchen and losing some sense of direction and control in the car."

"Her reactions are slower?"

"I would say so."

"Do you think she should think about not driving?"

"Do you want to be the one to suggest it? She drives better than half the drivers out there. It isn't her driving — steering and braking — that have slipped as much as her sense of loca- tion. She's a little unsure about where she is. She misses turns until she's on top of them. She thinks I miss off-ramps because she sees cars ahead go off, so we should go off too. This is on roads she knows well. Mostly it's in the kitchen that I'm aware of things not going in the usual way. I don't know quite how to explain it. She seems at times not to see the whole picture with all its implications. She sees only a part of what's going on."

"Damon told us," Marion said.

"Well, Damon isn't a bad witness."

Jerry asked, "Do you think something in the back of her mind might be bothering her? Does Stella ever seem depressed?"

"No, nothing like that. The best I can describe it is that sometimes she stops dead and seems to become introspective. Her demeanor is not depressed. It is more like resting. I notice it when she practices. I'm used to hearing a certain regularity and steadiness. Her attention seems to wander. She gets off the page and kind of daydreams."

"Is she aware of the kinds of thing you're talking about? Does she talk about it?"

"She knows she isn't walking right. She knows her memory is slipping, and I try to be reassuring about that. As for the car and the kitchen and other things, I'm honestly not sure how aware she is. She doesn't like to have it called to her attention."

"She's going to see her doctor?"

"I'll have to get that done."

"How about you? Is this keeping you up nights?"

"I'm fine."

"Think about yourself. You have to take care of yourself." There was a momentary pause while I thought he was waiting for me to say something. He said, "You're Stella's number one."

I was to hear "Take care of yourself" often after that. It is what you say to the spouse.

COMING in from the garden to a darkened house late in an overcast afternoon, I went through the house calling for her quietly. Not a light was on. If she was napping I didn't want to wake her. I found her in the bathroom, standing at the mirror in dark twilight.

What was she doing?

She said she was dressing. She seemed confused. I asked if she had been napping.

"A little," she said.

"Do you know what time it is?" I switched on the light so she could read her watch.

"It's a quarter to six."

I had a suspicion. "Morning or evening?"

"Morning."

When I told her it was evening, dinnertime, she didn't get it. We went into the kitchen and she had a bowl of cereal. I counted on finding something in the fridge to warm up. She gradually became convinced it was evening by the programs on TV. It wasn't a matter of changing her mind. She simply ceased to exist in morning mode and moved to evening mode.

"You've been a little off," I said. "Your chemistry may be out of whack. Maybe there's a pill you ought to know about. I'm going to call Loughrand in the morning and make an appointment for you." Stella did not resist at all.

Loughrand's secretary booked her and I followed up by sending a note without Stella's knowledge:

> When you see Stella please consider that something is going on that seems to be occasional disorientation of time and location. You might not notice it in an ordinary interview as her social presence is normal.
>
> She seems occasionally to lose a sense of the process she is in. It isn't simple old-age forgetfulness like forgetting appts, misplacing glasses, etc. We expect that.

Examples: Not sure whether we have had March or is it next month. Confuses in/out, back/front, up/down, left/right, morning/evening.

Does a lot of what I would call daydreaming. Sitting without occupation. No evident depression at all.

Losing natural athletic competence in driving a car. Has to think of what to do next. Where to stop the lever when she takes it out of park. Etc.

Also walking somewhat infirmly. She saw Kelley last month. He says her hip replacements are OK.

I am concerned that this may be an effect of small strokes we don't know about. Stella seldom has headaches. One or two aspirin clear them.

Please treat this as your own initiative without implicating me. I am reluctant to seem to be going around Stella in any way — including writing this note without telling her. I don't want to alarm her but I want to be sure to alert you.

Rereading that letter four years later, I am humbled to have been that obtuse. I wanted to be on top of the problem early. I was already late. I not only did not mention Alzheimer's to Loughrand as a possibility, I had not even thought of it until Stella and I were in the car on the way to his office.

BEFORE taking medical questions to doctors I vet them in the *Merck Manual*. In 1994 I upgraded to the *Merck Manual of Geriatrics* and considered myself as current as a layman needed to be. Not that I understand very much medical jargon or expect to one-up a professional who has gone to graduate schools and practiced medicine to the verge of retirement, but I come out of *Merck* with some education in symptoms and false symptoms, the probable course of treatment, the basic terms in which the patient's complaint will be discussed.

In the days before Stella's appointment I went into *Merck* at "Stroke," thrashed around in "Cardiovascular," and shifted to "Neurologic Disorder" where I was led, reference by reference, through the thicket of closely written, well-indexed pages, to "Senile Dementia of the Alzheimer Type." I know now, having read many books and technical papers, that in *Merck*'s dozen tightly written pages from "Normal Aging and Patterns of Neurologic Disease" through "SDAT" are about all the facts any layperson has to know of Alzheimer's. The facts, not the experience. Alzheimer's is not only what it is medically, it is a warren of unexpected nuances that those who have been caregivers try to prepare others for.

Until that first look into *Merck,* Alzheimer's was not even in my working vocabulary. I read about Algeria with more attention than I gave to Alzheimer's. If asked to spell it I would have gone down.

Merck did not persuade me that "Senile Dementia of the Alzheimer's Type" had anything to do with Stella. To the contrary, the very word "dementia" was ludicrous for the essentially normal woman Stella was. Dementia was insanity. Dementia went straight to Abraham Lincoln pointing at the brick wall of the asylum and telling his poor wife she would end there if she didn't shape up.

The first words of the crucial paragraph were, "The early stage of SDAT is characterized by recent memory loss . . ." If that was an essential characteristic, whatever was happening to Stella must be something else. I kept reverting to the questions: What is recent about knowing how to drive a car? What is recent about knowing how to scramble an egg?

I did not read very carefully then what I came back to later: the disease is characterized by an "inability to learn and retain new information, language problems, lability of mood." (How many days and hours of unexpected turns of behavior are embraced in those three words — lability of mood!) There may be "changes in personality. Patients may have progressive difficulty performing activities of living (e.g., balancing their checkbook, finding their way around, or remembering where they put things)."

Merck warned that the disease would go its own rogue way, symptoms would appear more or less aggressively at different times and from case to case, not in strict progression or relationship. In one victim there might never be the "paranoia, depression and agitation" that ravaged another. In its early stages Alzheimer's might "not compromise sociability. Patients may be alert, making it difficult for the practitioner to uncover problems of cognition." And ultimately, "SDAT is not curable."

None of this impressed me as having anything to do with Stella, inasmuch as she had not, at the threshold test of short-term memory loss, qualified for this incurable, brain-destroying disease that could be masked by normal social behavior so that even doctors might not recognize it.

It did not occur to me that what medical professionals mean by short-term memory is different from what you and I mean. We think of real events in real lives. They think of the patient's ability to recall a specific series of words after a short delay. Paper. Table. Barn. Airplane. Five minutes later: Now can you tell me those four words? The test seemed to me too elementary to be significant. As I learned, it had one virtue: it worked.

On the morning of Stella's visit to Loughrand, the vogue word for my state of mind was "denial." Dumb is more exact.

In its laconic way *Merck* mentioned a "Serial Sevens" test as a marker for Alzheimer's without stating what the test was. Presumably a professional reader would know. *Merck*'s reference recalled to me a magazine article I had read that described a Sevens test even simpler than the Word Recall test. I thought I must have missed something. Damon would have suspected a trick and ransacked every word for hidden meaning. On the way to the appointment with Loughrand, Sevens popped into my head, and I said to Stella, "Here's an arithmetic test for you. It starts — are you ready?—subtract seven from a hundred."

She didn't answer. Did she think there was a catch? "Go ahead — seven from a hundred."

She answered tentatively, "Eighty-eight?"

Math was not as tightly wrapped into Stella as it is in many musicians, but she had a graduate degree in business and had kept our checkbook for many years when I was too impatient to keep a running tally with which to contest the bank's monthly statement. I allowed a moment for her to reconsider. She did not.

"Here's the next step. Take away (the language of our childhood) seven from ninety-three."

Again the hesitation. When the answer came it was in the realm of magic, of incantation, not arithmetic. "Eighty-three? No, eighty-four?" A fuse seemed to blow. "Seventy-eight?"

My foot lagged off the accelerator as if to delay thinking the unthinkable. I saw with slow clarity that my wife whose hand I reached for had an inexorably wasting, incurable affliction of which she had no knowledge. I wanted to stay on this pleasant country road and the long circling drive around the marsh that would bring us back to Dr. Loughrand's when I was better composed.

"Close enough," I said.

We were at Loughrand's driveway sign and I turned in.

2

The New Primary Care Physician

At your tenth high-school reunion many of your cadre had already gone down — down at Birth, Scarlet Fever, Mumps, Measles, Mastoiditis, Flu, Diphtheria, Snake Bite, Giving Birth, War, Polio, Industrial Accident, Automobile Fatality — the innumerable hazards of living.

New cadres joined the game each year. Some words on the list were not proposed as often: childhood diseases were discarded almost entirely, some erased by antibiotics, some by inoculation. In their places are difficult new words: AIDS, Drive-by Gunfire.

You are in pretty good shape. At your fiftieth reunion the main challenges remaining seem to be cancer and cardiovascular disease — and for these, second chances for good behavior are often given: Exercise! Avoid saturated fats! Breathe deep! Practice yoga! Stop worrying! and you may reach the rewards of old age in good health and enjoy a quiet passing.

You begin to hear a word you have not thought much about: Alzheimer's. It has rarely been proposed to your contemporaries. It is out there for people in their late sixties and seventies and beyond. Alzheimer's? How do you spell it? The medical establishment must be getting a handle on it. It will be removed from the list. Like Polio. Like Measles. But it's still there.

In the long run, Alzheimer's may be the only word you have to get right. They don't yet have a handle on it, and there are no second chances. The Alzheimer's Association, which keeps track of these things, says if you are sixty-five, look around: one out of every ten people your age and older will get Alzheimer's. If you make it to eighty-five, the probability becomes one in two.

Think about that. People are living longer. If you expect to make it to eighty-five, expect also that you or your spouse will have Alzheimer's, the other will be a caregiver. Stella and I did not beat the odds.

I SHOULD have gone into Loughrand's examining room with Stella, but I had not since her first pregnancy gone with her beyond a waiting room. Some of it may have been the reticence of our generation, and more was respect that we had for each other's individuality, but mostly it was habit. I would not have expected her to come with me to my urologist while I discussed my prostate, but neither did we go together to the dentist, where there was no more an issue of privacy than at the barber's or the beauty shop that we also visited separately. Inside the walls of our house Stella and I were as contemporary as our children. After visits to doctors we routinely expected full disclosure and gave it.

Not since that half hour with Loughrand has Stella seen a doctor without me in a chair beside her. I am there to see that a busy opthalmologist does not unintentionally bully her into saying this is clearer than that before she is fully satisfied with her choice. Hairline differences may not matter to him, but in that case why ask? Now that she cannot stand at the camera but must be X-rayed lying down, I sit with her for the two hours it sometimes takes to get properly mammogrammed. I'm there while the lab assistant takes three tubes of blood and when Loughrand scopes her sigmoid and swabs her cervix. I am there to remember how long ago her hip joints were replaced, what allergies she has, how much time she gives the treadmill, at what speed. How often does she urinate? Does she have trouble falling asleep? How many glasses of water does she drink every day? And, lately, to confirm how many grandchildren she has. It becomes a little nebulous where children end and grandchildren begin.

I walk the line between Stella wanting me to remember for her and the interrogator wanting her to remember. I am prepared to back out if I suspect he thinks my presence may inhibit her answers to bedroom questions or questions about her interior life, but I don't doubt that Stella wants me to stay; and

I do stay (except at the dentist's — I have never been in a dentist's office laid out conducively to third-party witnesses).

My intentions may deserve her trust, but I continually question my performance. I have never gotten all the way past the realization that I could have seen many months — maybe years — sooner that it was not merely aging, it was Alzheimer's that had hold of her. If I had seen sooner, she would have been on medication sooner, but I knew nothing about that then.

While I sat in Loughrand's waiting room that day, thinking about the damn Sevens, I gave myself the test and had no difficulty running it down into the forties, as far as I had the introspective patience for it. Questions occurred: In the same way, could Stella ask *herself* and get it right? If it were in *writing* would she get it right?

Loughrand came to the waiting room door only long enough to tell me that my wife was in good physical shape. You can't always read this stout, furry, reticent man behind his beard and glasses. He said around the door jamb that he had "some ideas" we should talk about when he had test results later in the week. In the meantime he had written her an order to take to the blood lab and another for a CT scan, both at the hospital. On the way home I asked her how things had gone.

"He says I'm in good shape. I told him about forgetting things. He asked me what he always asks: was I having headaches? I said yes, I had one-aspirin headaches now and then but not often. He said he'd like me to get a scan. It's a precaution for anybody my age who gets headaches."

"What's he looking for?"

"The headaches and at least some of the forgetfulness may be from small strokes I'm not even aware of. A lot of people get them and never know it. He doesn't think anything is there but he wants to be sure. He asked me a lot of dumb questions."

"Give him the benefit of the doubt. He has his reasons. What questions?"

"How old I am, what is my birthday, what year was I born. It's all in his records. With computers everywhere I didn't think they had to ask the same questions over and over. Would you believe I couldn't remember the year I was born?"

"If you say so. Did you get it right eventually?"

She was canny. "When was I born?"

"Nineteen fourteen, the same year I was."

"That's what I thought." He had puzzled her. "He wanted to know if I knew what county I live in. Did I ever know what county I lived in? The last word I know that went with county was Allegheny."

"Pittsburgh is in Allegheny County. The last time you lived there was almost fifty years ago, right after the War." (We had only one war, World War II; the rest needed defining.)

"I remember that. Allegheny County, PA."

"Do you remember the name of the county you lived in in New Jersey?"

Not a chance.

"You were treasurer of the women's shelter. You must have written the county name a hundred times." She didn't have it. It was forty years ago. I gave it to her.

"Where would they get a name like Middlesex? It wasn't the thing to be then. Nobody cares anymore. He asked me to name the president before Kennedy. A lot of things I know perfectly well I can't say on demand. I always preferred multiple-choice tests."

Information is an overvalued commodity (compared, for example, to good judgment, kindness, honesty, persistence, and other virtues not in oversupply), and I don't know why it should distress anybody not to be able to recall names that are no longer useful to know. It is, however, an expected social grace to have the names of historical figures, as it is to have the names of countries and common flowers, and the name of a recent president happened to be one of the bits and pieces, individually not of much point, which collectively gave Loughrand his diagnosis that something in Stella's memory was not working. I gave her the name of the president before Kennedy.

"I know that! Do you think Dr. Loughrand doesn't think I know Eisenhower was president?"

"On a multiple-choice you would have gotten it."

"That's what I mean. Questions don't find out what you know. He asked me to spell words backward. Does anybody know a word any better because he can spell it backward? Can you spell words backward?"

"Give me one."

She gave me "World." I can't say I snapped it out but I read it printed in the air. I explained, "They have records that tell them how thousands of people answer those questions. They find a norm. If you deviate from a norm it gives them something to think about."

"Suppose I forgot Eisenhower, suppose I remembered it was Nixon. Would I have a mental problem?"

"I don't know, Stell. If you said Napoleon you might have a mental problem. Based on experience, they have expectations."

We continued to talk after we got home. In the envelope with orders for the blood lab and the hospital scan was a page with a printout of a clock face with the hands at 8:20 and the legend DRAW THIS CLOCK. On a second page was a childish drawing of a clock face at about 10:45. I could not imagine that Stella had drawn it. It was the kind of drawing young mothers post on refrigerator doors. The numbers were skewed to the upper left quadrant of a circle. The circle had a caved-in right side. The distortion suggested a Picasso face deconstructed to more than the one plane to which flat canvas confines an artist's imagination. It was as if Stella had seen the face from the front and in profile in one glance.

"What's this all about?"

"I was supposed to copy the clock. I can't draw freehand circles."

Both pages may have been folded into the envelope by mistake, although I guessed that Loughrand in sidelong mode intended me to see them.

"Did he ask you to subtract seven from a hundred?"

She wasn't sure. "Something like that. There were so many questions I was confused. He asked me to look at things on the floor and remember what I saw and then tell him."

"What about sevens? If you tell doctors you're forgetting things they're supposed to ask if you can subtract seven from a hundred."

"You want me to give you the answer?"

"If you feel like it."

She gave me ninety-one.

"Let's see something." I got a sheet of paper and under 100 wrote − 7. "Now try."

She took a few seconds and wrote 93. I entered −7 under the sum and asked her to subtract. She struggled again and got 86. She was able to work out on paper what she couldn't figure in her head. Oral and written — different memory paths.

I am long past the belief that I had an insight the doctors didn't about the nature of memory loss in the early stage of Alz. It remains true that long-practiced habits — driving, cooking, brushing teeth, and tying shoelaces — are also forgotten; but if repetition of the Sequential Sevens twice within an hour did not diminish its diagnostic usefulness, it is evidence that loss of short-term memory is Alzheimer's striking characteristic.

I went to the library to augment *Merck*. The two standard consumer medical books on the reference shelf, with the same publication year, 1994, as *Merck,* had so little information that a reader would have been neither alerted nor informed. On the circulating shelves were titles that looked like better possibilities. I took them to a carrel to scan texts, compare copyright dates, and read enough pages to decide what to carry home. At the pharmacy I got the information sheet on tacrine, the generic name of the only drug then cleared by the FDA for open Alzheimer's prescription.

By the end of the week when Loughrand's secretary called me to come in I was a layman well-informed on diseases that cause memory disorders and gloomily sure I was looking at Alzheimer's.

LOUGHRAND would not have had a blood chemistry report that said *Alzheimer's*. It can't be read in the blood. The CT scan he had ordered would not image the tangle of nerves and sludge of dead cells that defines Alz; they were then beyond the instrument's vision until the patient died and the pathologist could safely enter the brain. Alz in the living was diagnosed from the patient's history and behavior — from symptoms, not source — and confirmed by process of elimination when the imaging scan did not find stroke.

Magnetic resonance and tomography imaging scans know stroke when they see it. If present, stroke may account for behavior that would otherwise be attributed to Alzheimer's.

Nor was she an alcohol or drug abuser. Her symptoms weren't the fringe of multiple sclerosis, delirium, glandular abnormality, depression, nutrition deficiency or a different, less common, mental disorder such as Pick's or Kreutzfeld-Jakob (England's mad cow disease).

All possibilities lingered — even the possibility that Stella was one of the "walking well" who, innocently or not, exhibited symptoms of illnesses they didn't have. But in practice, if the scan did not find a stroke trail, the plausibility of Alz came center stage. The rest stayed in the diagnostician's reserve until in time their plausibility faded to nothing. If it is not stroke, cases with similar symptoms in persons of advanced age are overwhelmingly Alz. Not in every case, but statistically it is powerfully persuasive.

Within its limited horizon the scan had found that Stella's brain was essentially healthy. Unfortunately, its horizon wasn't broad enough to include the areas of dissolution. Loughrand said, "We are left with an inference that something outside the view of the CT is the cause of the derangement."

I did not like *derangement* any more than I had liked *dementia* and I remain unpersuaded by arguments from linguistics, etymology, philology, semiology, or other constructs that do not take account of the way ordinary people react to ordinary words. When the first publicity appeared about a new research facility to be built in Washington, it stated that the primary focus will be on Alzheimer's and it will be named the Dementia Center. *Dementia Center* is a choice as obtuse as an older generation's *Lunatic Asylum*.

EVEN before the scan, Loughrand was entitled to a gut conclusion. Our part of the world attracts retired senior citizens, and

Loughrand had given many of the elders in his waiting room the same selective questions from the Mental State Inpatient Consultation Form, summarized in *Merck,* that he gave Stella. He had seen enough Picasso clocks, heard enough sevens and words spelled backward and misremembered names of objects, birthdays, and presidents to be reasonably sure that brain scans and elaborate examinations by neurologists and psychiatrists would in the end see what he saw in an office visit.

He said, "I hoped the CT would tell us what we prefer to hear." I did not like the idea that stroke was preferable to its alternatives. "We have to consider other sources of dementia."

I did not like anything I heard but I had been prepared to hear it. I did not give him the benefit of my lay diagnosis based on a few days of selective reading, and Loughrand had some housekeeping to do before he stated an opinion. He mainly had to dispose of depression. A definable disease, not merely a state of mind, depression is sometimes mistaken for Alz and often coexists with it. Like Alzheimer's, depression does not present as an emergency; unlike Alzheimer's, depression has a battery of treatment options.

"Is Stella depressed about anything? About her condition?" He recited a list cursorily: melancholia? she sleeps well? any weight loss? lethargy? He did not look at me for a sign of concealment. He had a checklist. He had his duty to ask, I to respond. Any family problems? Any recent change in her demeanor?

There had been no change. She had always had a level temperament and still did, except that she barked at me if she thought I was nannying her.

"This daydreaming you mention in your letter?"

"It isn't dour. It is more nearly — resting. More nearly — absent from the table."

I lingered on my description of her demeanor when she daydreamed. When asked what was on her mind she answered, "Nothing, really." Loughrand looked at his papers. He had asked her these questions. He was getting a second opinion.

"Any unexplained crying episodes?"

She had cried only once in recent months that I knew of, and it was from physical injury when she fell. A few tears had leaked out while she clasped her arm that would the next morning be violently colored. She had never been much of a crying person. In recent months I had not noticed her taking out a handkerchief even during touching episodes in movies. She was more likely to doze.

"No profound and continuing grief?"

"Nothing like that."

"No occasion for it or not that kind of response?"

She had not cried to hear that her longest-lived friend, going all the way back to grade school, had died. After she said she was sorry to hear it and hung up, she said, "Mary Canaday died this morning in her bed. Heart failure. That's too bad," and apparently cleared it from her mind. In Loughrand's office I lingered again at the equanimity with which she had heard the end of Mary Canaday, but Loughrand had asked about more grief, not less, and I was not there to chat.

Loughrand went on down his list. "She has no hand tremor. We can rule out Parkinson's. How much alcohol does she drink?" Like depression, alcoholism can briefly be mistaken for Alz.

"In a big week maybe two light glasses of wine. She always shows you the measure of what she wants — an inch. If we go to a party she may take a vodka and tonic. 'Very easy on the vodka.' I've never known her to take two."

"To your knowledge were either of her parents or grand-parents or any older relatives what you might regard as senile in old age? Did they need nursely companions? Did they live their last years in what were called 'homes'? You get the bearing of the question?"

Stella had not come to me with a lot of relatives, and the few I knew had died of cancer and cardiac involvement. In their eighties Stella's parents had gotten around well until the same familiar terminal incidents. Stella's sister, a few years older, was in bright mental health, and remained so until pneumonia took her two years after Stella's Alz was diagnosed. If it was genetic, Stella was a narrow target in a family that was not passing the disease down.

From what I had read, scientists were not on the hot trail of anything curative, nothing that reversed the disease, but they had well in view a way to alter a chromosome so that many potential Alz cases — maybe half they said in the early nineteen nineties, but later they cut the estimate sharply — would never occur. Genetic alteration might have something to do with her unborn great-grandchildren, not Stella.

Stella's family history left him silent. He was uncomfortable as he moved toward disclosing the necessary conclusion to the patient's husband. Diagnosis and prescription are professionally satisfying, but a disease that is all downhill without even pain to mitigate by prescription offers little professional reward.

I said, "I'm trying to get the whole picture. She isn't an alcoholic. She doesn't get depressed. It isn't stroke. What else can it be?"

"I'm considering prescribing Cognex," he said. "Before we do that we should consult on it with a neurologist."

"Isn't Cognex the brand name of tacrine?"

"Yes."

"And that's specific for Alzheimer's?"

"Well, not only for Alzheimer's — but yes." He stopped scratching his beard and seemed to enlarge in his chair. It was the first time the word had been uttered between us and he was visibly relieved that it came from me. We were up to prescriptions and monitoring the patient's progress, services he was comfortable with.

ALL week I had put off talking to the children and tonight was the night.

"Oh man," Damon said, "Does Mom know?"

"She knows something isn't right inside her, but it isn't painful and she doesn't think of it as something that won't go away. She knows she isn't walking well, but as far as she is concerned it could be arthritis acting up or something that goes back to her hip replacements. It's more fretful than earth-shaking to her."

"Does she talk about how she feels?"

"Not much, and I don't ask more than she would usually expect. I don't want to alarm her. I judge her mood and act accordingly. I'm pretty good at that."

"You're going to get a second opinion?"

"Loughrand says he will refer me to a neurologist but I haven't committed. He'll be one of the hospital crowd and I have mixed feelings. I might prefer to see somebody in Boston. I want your input and Connie's, and your sister's and Jerry's." That covered the children and their spouses, every one informed and thoughtful; we all consulted back and forth on many subjects.

"I'll get Connie on the other line. She'll have better questions than mine."

Our daughter-in-law is the director of professional personnel at a teaching hospital in Massachusetts. She can find out with a phone call who the top doctors are. She can mine the literature in the hospital library. She and Stella have always gotten along fine. She is emotionally in it for Stella.

"Dad, I'm so sorry to hear this. You know, this is a disease there is no way to be absolutely sure of. They can't see well enough into the brain —"

"I'm up on that. I've learned a lot in the past couple of days. I've read everything in our public library on it. I know they can see the plaques and tangles in the brain only after the patient dies and there is an autopsy. But by elimination they get to a working hypothesis."

"Is it your family physician who says Alzheimer's? What is he, internal medicine?"

"Yes. We have an elderly population around here. He sees a lot of people and I'm satisfied he's a good observer."

"Probably so, but you'll want to see a neurologist."

"I want to think it through. I feel fairly well-educated in this. I wanted to talk first to the family."

"Have you talked to Marion?"

"After we hang up."

"Marion is near Johns Hopkins. It's a big subject there. She may not know that. She is near the National Institutes for Health, too. There would be a lot going on there. Marion will know how to go about it. I'll call her. In the meantime, I'll pull some photocopies from the hospital library and get a packet to you. And Dad, you have to think about yourself. You have to take care of yourself, too. Alzheimer's is a long-distance race."

When Stella had appendicitis and broke a hip and broke another hip, nobody told me I had to take care of myself. There must be an instinct about the exhaustion of Alzheimer care.

I brought Marion and Jerry up-to-date. Marion didn't know about Johns Hopkins but she would find out who was connected there. She knew how to use the National Institutes of Health. Otherwise, she and Jerry had the same concerns as Connie and Damon. They had the same questions and ended with the same admonition: take care of yourself.

An hour after Marion hung up she was on the phone again. There was somebody I should talk to. Carey Dingman was expecting my call. It didn't make any difference how late. Yes, she had spoken to Connie. They were on track. Call Carey. Carey was a family counselor, a consultant to Marion's agency, a psychologist with big credentials who had chosen to have a rural practice. Carey was hands-on. He made house visits. He knew many cases of Alzheimer's. He was a wise old man, not as old as her father but close enough (and wiser). We would get along.

While I dialed Carey Dingman I became worried that I would become overloaded and have conflicting priorities. I didn't think we would be going to Washington, D.C. Maybe Boston, but that was only a two-hour drive. When my father had heart trouble he had been referred by his GP in Pittsburgh to the care of a doctor at a hospital in New York City. What had the GP been thinking when he sent an eighty-year-old man and woman (of course, my mother would not stay behind) to live for three months in a hotel around the corner from the sainted cardiologist and his shrine of a hospital, far from friends and family and the conveniences of their own home and neighborhood, while a half mile from their front door was a great medical conglomerate of specialists and hospitals clustered around the University of Pittsburgh? If there were not talent and facilities enough around the university, ten minutes by car across the river was another equally impressive medical complex.

At the time I had muted my rage at what seemed to me to be thoughtless doctoring that trafficked only in diseases and disregarded the people to whom diseases happened; I had not wanted my parents to lose confidence in the care they were getting.

I had reason to reserve enthusiasm for the hospital and certain specialties in our own much smaller part of the world, but that did not imply alternatives in New York or Washington. Boston was within reason. I did not then know how little doctoring there is to Alzheimer's, but I was mentally prepared to drive in every morning to access the renowned medical services of Boston if I could have Stella back within familiar walls by night.

"Carey Dingman here."

From a suburb of Washington, D.C. where I did not intend to go, he came right through, already a friend. He was across the table. I told him Marion said it wouldn't be too late to call. "Anytime for Marion. You have a fine daughter, Aaron. You are a lucky man. I would do anything I can for her. She does so much for others."

I said I didn't know what could be done over the phone, but Marion thought it would be useful if we talked.

"Let us see if we can justify ourselves to Marion. Your family physician thinks your wife probably has Alzheimer's?" He asked me to spell Loughrand. "Loughrand has seen a scan and rules out stroke?"

That's where we were as of that morning.

"Has he known Stella a long time? Does he see her often?"

For twenty years he has seen her for her annual checkup, for her flu shot, and another once or twice a year for whatever came up.

"So she isn't a stranger. Marion says you're a good reader and have been reading about the disease. What have you been reading?"

On the table beside me were *Alzheimer's Disease: A Guide for Families* by Powell and Courtice, *The 36-Hour Day* by Mace and Rabins, *Understanding Alzheimer's* by Aronson. Aronson had some kind of connection with Johns Hopkins.

"Tell your library to protect its copy of Aronson. It's either out of print or out of stock."

I didn't think Loughrand would have known anything like that. I had looked at the library copy and decided I wanted to own it, and only that morning, after making a call to its wholesale supplier, the bookstore said it wasn't available.

"Do you think Loughrand has diagnosed it right?"

I was not qualified to judge right or wrong. I accepted Loughrand's diagnosis because it was plausible and conformed to what I saw myself.

Carey asked me to give him some "for instances" of what I had observed in Stella. He asked me how long did I think Stella had had a problem before I recognized it. I told him it might have been as much as six months, a year. What did Loughrand think the next step should be? He had proposed that Stella see a neurologist for a second opinion.

"Your hospital has a new center for psychiatric disorders. Do you know about it?"

Loughrand had not mentioned it.

"You may want to look into it. Psychiatry is an alternate route to a second opinion and is often simpler. Psychiatry relies essentially on an observation of the patient and a battery of question-and-answer tests. Neurology has more instrumental tests. Nobody can ever say finally that it's Alzheimer's or it isn't, but at a certain point you have a working answer and you go with it. Nothing is lost if you are a little premature or even wrong. Something may be lost by delay."

So — Stella's situation might be more urgent than I had supposed?

"In this way, if it's Alzheimer's, you have to get yourself set for a decline over months, over years. With tacrine the rate of decline may be slowed. It may not be a great drug, but many drugs that don't work very well late in the course of a disease are effective in its earlier stages. It follows logically, doesn't it, that the sooner tacrine is administered, the more likely it is to arrest decline at a higher level of well-being."

I was already a year late and proceeding at leisure. I felt the weight of failed responsibility. I did not need to discuss that with Carey. He was not my confessor. We were at *now*. "So what are you saying? That we should get the fastest diagnosis and begin medication as soon as we can?"

Instead of answering me, he had a question of his own: Did I have absolute faith in Loughrand?

I didn't have absolute faith in any doctor. I would distrust a doctor who demanded it. Loughrand was not that kind of man at all. His orders were like suggestions of things that might work in an environment of conjecture and uncertainty. "Let's see how this goes," he would say, handing me tubes and packets from his sample box. "Try these." Rather than grill me about my complaints, he heard me out in the examining room and retired to his back office, I assumed to commune with a text. When he came back he spoke for the book into a neutral space and I was welcome to overhear. In my appointment times he never asked about Stella; it was as if he thought we might have separated or that she might have passed on since the last visit, something too painful to discuss.

Still, Loughrand was a thoughtful man and I listened to him carefully. He had been around a long time. I liked the way he went back over the ground with his stethoscope when he didn't get it the first time. A magazine article stated on impressive authority that half the new gatekeepers had no idea what they were listening for when they passed their stethoscopes over their patients and urged them to breathe deeply. It was just something doctors did. I was sure Loughrand knew. He was, at least by that measure, better than half the doctors.

I said, "I wouldn't follow him over the edge of a cliff, but I am comfortable with his judgments."

"It might be helpful if you thought of yourself as the physician and Loughrand as somebody you respect enough to consult with on major decisions. That's what most Alzheimer's cases wind up looking like."

I was the primary physician?

"Alzheimer's is not usually a doctor-intensive disease. It's more aide-and-caregiver intensive. There may be a doctor of record when they ask who your physician is, but much of the job will be yours. You will need advice from Dr. Loughrand, and your wife will see him — you will refer her to him when it is appropriate. But you will probably be in the driver's seat for most initiatives."

It was an idea to get used to. I had a start — I already felt that I had a relationship with the *Merck Manual.*

"When Stella's medical needs seem to be beyond your competence you will refer her to a specialist as Loughrand would. Loughrand would be her resource for internal and general family medicine. After you get a second opinion on the diagnosis, she might never have to see anybody outside the usual circle of dentistry, hearing, and sight. Maybe a podiatrist. Most people are used to booking those specialties direct."

"That's how we've always done it."

"All right, then. After the first flurry of diagnosis there may be very little medically to do. Alzheimer's is not a disease that responds to surgery or massive medication. There are no drug options. The medical requirements can be met by an infirmary on an Indian reservation if it's staffed by a caring person who reads a few books. That sounds almost like a layman, doesn't it? Somebody like you? The caregiver is the main person for Alzheimer's. It's a caregiver's disease more than a physician's."

"Do physicians know that?"

I had in mind a close friend who had a pacemaker installed by a surgeon recommended by his family doctor. When a discomfort developed before his scheduled follow-up, he called the surgeon who was not immediately available. The office referred the patient to an associate who, after discussing the symptoms on the phone, thought the problem was not cardiac but digestive. He referred the patient back to his family doctor. The family doctor, who had treated him and his family for ten years, told my friend he was no longer a patient; he had consulted another doctor — not the surgeon, to whom the referral had originally been made but the surgeon's associate — without speaking first to him. Some doctors had a high huff quotient. I had never seen that in Loughrand. Loughrand was my doctor. I listened to him. I didn't always take his advice and he didn't push. I didn't know any doctor or anybody else who was due unquestioned obedience. I thought I had some responsibilities other than to obey. There are a lot of people — doctors and others — out there testing how much leaning on you they can get away with. That wasn't Loughrand.

Loughrand had few certitudes. Occasionally I went to a specialist without a referral and when I told Loughrand he seemed relieved that the responsibility was mine. We hadn't "chosen" Loughrand. We inherited him when our doctor retired and sold his practice. It worked out all right.

These conversations were taking place before the sudden onset of the tide of managed care. When Stella was diagnosed, HMOs, especially in the East and outside the big cities, hardly existed for the elderly. Unless in the retirement program of a big corporation, we seniors were probably covered by Medicare or Medicaid. The catalog of errors in managed care practice that soon had to be addressed had its origin in the sudden appearance in force of a new way to practice medicine devised by people whose interest was investment opportunity. The commodity they sold was professional time, the less it cost them the better. I asked, "What does the primary care physician do that I may not know about?"

"He knows a lot about what kind of people you are, your lifestyle, your circumstances —" I knew that about Stella better than Loughrand did.

"He knows the limits of his own practice and refers the patient to the appropriate specialist when that is indicated. He keeps track of the case."

Who could do that better than I? Although doctors who practiced in outlying towns in our county seldom were hospital staff, they were often "courtesy staff" and their referrals were to staff. I once compared the gastroenterology assets of our hospital, which advertised itself to be "One of the 100 Best Hospitals in America" with one of the major teaching hospitals in Boston. The local staff was three board-certified men practicing all branches of the specialty. The Boston hospital had twenty-six board-certified gastroenterologists, most of them qualified in sub-specialties confined to the few inches of digestive tract where the patient's problem might actually exist. I had a bias toward local practices for many commonsense reasons, but I might more readily than Loughrand look elsewhere if I felt the need of a master whose practice was in inches, and not yards.

Dingman said that most experienced primary care doctors knew the practical considerations in an Alzheimer's case well enough and accepted a larger than usual amount of caregiver initiative.

"These are patients who month-to-month aren't getting well, either from medication or the healing power of time. From a medical viewpoint the symptoms are picayune, not the kind of thing doctors deal with in detail. The patient isn't eating, he's incontinent, she loses her glasses, his eyes are red, she hears whistling, she gets up at two in the morning and walks around, she takes off her shoes in restaurants and forgets them. It's a disease of numerous small daily events. A physician easily loses track of the status of a patient like that. A physician functions in his office. The parameters of his expectations are on his bookshelf or in the back of his mind, not in anecdotal information from patients. He is accustomed to the cycle of illness, treatment, and cure for particular problems. People make appointments for next week or next month. Alzheimer's doesn't lend itself to such expectations. Consider yourself lucky if Loughrand pays attention when you call him and is available when you need him. Do you have an Alzheimer's Association office near you?"

I didn't know. I had seen the association mentioned in books. While Carey told me what the association was I opened the directory and found a county listing a few towns up the road.

"I'd suggest you go in and talk to them and hear what they have to say before you make any final decisions about second opinions. They have literature you may find helpful. They should know the diagnostic resources."

We talked for the better part of an hour. I had never before been on the phone that long with anybody. We talked about the physical layout of our house, our financial resources, the cost of different kinds of care, my relationship with Stella and others in the family. He gave me new perspectives on the urgency of medication, the rhythm of the disease, the role of doctors. He called my attention to the hospital's psychiatric facility. He hadn't said demented.

Carey Dingman is a psychiatrist. I had invested years of resistance to psychiatry as I had to counseling, but Carey turned me around. It was again the never-quite-learned lesson that there are no professions, no trades, no sexes, races, or colors; there are only individuals who fill their places well or not-so-well.

At the end, after inviting me to call anytime, he said, "I'd be glad to see you, if you like, but you want to concentrate on finding what you need closer to home. Alzheimer's is not all that complicated medically. You don't have to wait for a confirming second opinion before taking your doctor's suggestion to get Stella on tacrine. The prescription name for that will be Cognex. If it's a false alarm, all right, discontinue the medication, no harm done at early dosage levels. Think hard about yourself. Unwind to as near a state of calm as you can and try to stay there. Remind yourself to feel a little Buddhistic regularly. Keep your blood pressure down. You may never have given thought to outliving your wife. Now you have to. Take care of yourself."

3

SECOND OPINIONS

AFTER A SECTION OF HIS colon was removed by a staff surgeon at a nearby hospital, a friend of mine continued to have bouts of severe pain that sent him back to the surgeon's office, on weekends to the hospital emergency room. He was assured everything was all right, those things took time. After a year without relief he signed himself into the emergency room of a major Boston hospital.

"They put me on a gurney and covered me with a sheet. The duty doctor called for a specialist. The specialist lifted the sheet and asked what seemed to be the trouble. While I told him about the operation a year ago and the pain he pressed his hand on my belly. He said to nobody in particular, 'Don't they know a hernia when they see one?'"

A second operation was scheduled and, as Dave Black told several of us not long after he came home, "That was all there was to it." Six years later he has not had a moment of pain after that agonizing year.

Most of us come to Alzheimer's with long memories of such medical experiences. The stories are disdained as "anecdotal evidence" and are compared to statistical records of professional success. However, what we ourselves have lived through or heard of color the way we think of doctors and hospitals. They become facts of the next experience.

The year I was slow to realize that Stella had crossed the threshold into Alzheimer's she and I were preoccupied by my sister Eve's cancer. When I realized at last what Stella was into and that I was her caregiver, I brought with me biases from Eve's last months.

Eve was younger than I by four years and widowed. After nominal retirement she still worked a full schedule of business consulting and community service. Stage by stage, test by test, procedure by procedure, Eve slipped in a few months from vigorous health to her death. She had been not only family but best friend for both Stella and me. She visited regularly from a time zone away; never more than a week without a phone call.

The beginning of Eve's illness, like Stella's, had been hardly worth noticing — a visit to a doctor for something women expect, an inconvenience, not an anxiety. There were lab tests, office procedures. Eve's gynecologist stepped her up to an oncologist of formidable reputation, master of a hospital team. A hysterectomy, described as routine in the circumstances for a woman of her age, followed. That during the operation they found cancer was less important than the good news that they thought they had gotten it all. Through the telephone I would have heard in the timbre of Eve's voice any disquiet she may have felt. She thought she was sailing through mildly adverse weather.

I didn't wake up until in another call she told me Dr. Skiles had ordered her back to the hospital and, in rapid sequence, that more cancer had been found and radiation therapy had begun.

I had not met Dr. Skiles. He had been identified for me one evening at the nurse's station where he had terrorized them on account of something one of them had not done by the book. I marked him down for rudeness, but at the same time it was in his favor that in a hospital of all places he had no tolerance for slack.

I made an appointment to meet him at his office, which was not grand, at the end of an anteroom full of patients. A half dozen of them were along one wall under domes re-mindful of a beauty salon; others sipped what looked like milkshakes. I thought there must be good reason for such an active practice in a city well-furnished with doctors attracted by two major medical schools and several major hospitals.

Skiles managed not only the surgery but also the medicine and the oncology of his patients, and while he did not site the beam and press the buzzer, the radiology technician's reports came directly to his desk. Associates from his office included Eve in their rounds, but she had seen no other physician of in-dependent weight. He went brusquely to the agenda before I was seated.

"You wished to see me about your sister."

I did not think he should see me as an adversary. I said there had been several disappointing outcomes for the doctor as well as the patient. I had no reason to think the management of her case was anything less than book-perfect, and I didn't want to suggest to Eve that the care she was receiving was in question, but all of us were only human, etc., etc. A consultation or second opinion would be timely. Didn't he agree it would be well to call in somebody — of his own choice — to consult?

No, he did not agree. "Anybody who knows anything will agree that the patient is being managed correctly."

"A reason to get another opinion is that it would be reassuring to my sister in what is a down period for her."

"It is not reassuring to your sister to put questions in her mind."

"I haven't discussed this with her. She is in a very tiring process and not up to making the kind of brisk decision she ordinarily makes. That's why I put it up to you."

"There is no point to calling anybody in. It's a waste of time and money. That was your question?" Short of calling in our seconds to agree on weapons, we were finished. I thought my sister would never knowingly put herself in the hands of such an imperious personality. Illnesses make their own decisions on their own timetables, seldom offering convenient options.

I put a call through to a family friend, a veteran of the National Cancer Institute, now practicing near New York City. He quizzed out of me what I knew and volunteered to call Skiles, explain the family connection, and talk it over.

In a couple of days he called back that Skiles seemed to be first-class. While the outcomes had been unhappy, it was the nature of cancer to not always fulfill the best expectations. I don't know whether it was to my satisfaction or regret that this family friend, who had the best training and led the oncology department of a university hospital, said he would probably have handled Eve's case the way Skiles did. Manners were something else — "Don't pay too much attention to manners. The doctor is there to practice medicine."

At about that time an argument erupted between Skiles and the hospital. He picked up his staff, patients, and big-league ball and went to another hospital, inconveniently located for the visits of Eve's friends. She said she had been asked if it was all right with her to be transferred and she had said yes. She had signed papers. It was all done in a day. Had I been there that day I might have said, "Stay here. The surroundings are familiar, you like the nurses, and friends can visit easily. There must be other physicians up to the job." Or I might not have. It is seldom convenient to make the right speech, especially from another time zone. In six weeks we buried my sister.

Skiles had been her physician for eight months. He had seen her go from almost well to bad to worse. It stays with me that he didn't call or send a note of condolence, didn't say a word of regret or closure to me or to Eve's son, also from a distant city — nobody lives near where they are needed anymore — who had been even more regularly attentive than I and had applied quicker intelligence to the numerous questions that came up in the course of his mother's illness.

"Forget it," said someone who had buried many family members. "Doctors don't send condolences after they lose patients."

If it's true, it supports my suspicion that often doctors don't treat patients, they treat the accepted profile of the patient's disease, not always the same thing.

When I tell the hernia story to laymen, their attention goes to the botched operation and the reluctance to admit it. I told it to a doctor. He winced and said, "Couldn't the Boston man have said a few noncommittal words and repaired the hernia without making a point of the botch?" I thought that, in a high-class way, that is what police did when a rogue cop shot up a neighborhood.

A MEDICAL column speaks in a warning voice, "Choose your doctor carefully." In ancient Araby such words had only to be uttered and the genie materialized. In the real world, choose how?

Ask the hospital. The response is the staff list. Is that all there is to it? A staff doctor did Dave Black's hernia.

There's a doctor in your church, temple, mosque, at your gym, in your fraternal society. Ask your friends. You may get positive reports based on limited experience: my father, a man of many enthusiasms, routinely referred to any doctor, barber, or therapist he had a good experience with (and, in fact, the man who shined his shoes) as "the best in the business."

You may get negative reports: a surgeon is bad-mouthed for taking out an innocent appendix when the patient had merely the fiery tension of cat scratch fever. You look it up in *Merck* and read that cat scratch fever, if left alone, may cure itself in six weeks or so. But in real life time is short, and peritonitis lurks more frequently than cats. Decisions have to be made, and symptoms that are usually reliable indicators of appendicitis result in the wrong call from a very good surgeon.

Physicians who are not up to speed don't call attention to themselves by pulling into the slow lane and blinking caution lights. Professionals — teachers, police, firefighters, doctors

— are collegial; if you were in the club they might speak to you more openly. How can I, essentially a stranger, be trusted with any more than Loughrand's prudentially stated warning that Dr. Remnant would not be his first choice to consult on a neurological matter? If, after walking around the block as gossip, the statement came back as, "Loughrand says Remnant should not be licensed," it could be an embarrassment. It could result in a letter from a lawyer.

Better that some unknown patient suffer in some unknown way than the doctor embarrass himself by blowing a whistle. (Who knows, Remnant may never kill anybody, he doesn't operate; he went to a good school; maybe he doesn't drink as much as he used to.) Truth-telling against the tribe is abhorrent.

Gingerly admitted by the profession to exist as a class, undesirables are harder to identify individually, and when we choose doctors we are looking for individuals.

More than most caregivers, I may have carried into my role of primary physician an attitude of reserve about things medical.

RIGHT now I had to settle on a doctor in General Practice to stay with while Alz made its run. That would probably be Loughrand. He already had the watch. I knew I could live with him.

I also had to settle on somebody else for a second opinion. Should I let Loughrand select the neurologist? We thought Loughrand a sound diagnostician, reassuringly conservative, perhaps not quite leading-edge enough on new medications. He didn't find it necessary to run the patient-cluttered waiting room thought of in the profession as the mark of successful practice. He was not difficult about seeing our minor emergencies or returning phone calls that accumulated over weekends.

What he lacked was what may be too much to expect of any doctor: a whole view of our medical lives and a sense of urgency that we ourselves felt about our aches and pains. He had no insistence in him, which implied not lack of professional competence but lack of sufficient conviction to want his advice to prevail; or it could be read as lack of deep concern. As you see, we subconsciously required Loughrand to walk several fine lines. Had he crossed one, we might have thought him arrogant.

It is not unusual that the match between patients and doctors, who may have inherited each other or met in an emergency or under the auspices of a long-cured disease, is not made in heaven. If it can be said of marriages in a country where the divorce rate is on the order of fifty percent it can certainly be said of medical relationships. I intended my new persona as primary physician to be more subtle than overt, more in my thinking than in Loughrand's practice. Stella and I would continue to have the essential aspect of regular patients. We still needed checkups and flu shots and papers of record executed; somebody to sound out and take counsel with, even if only as a point of departure; somebody to get started with as he had just got us started on Alzheimer's.

After Carey Dingman I knew I had more options than the neurologist at the other end of Loughrand's phone. I didn't know how good the options were but I had them. Dingman had mentioned the psychiatric facility at our hospital. He had mentioned the Alzheimer's Association.

Loughrand didn't know he had been displaced by an amateur, and it was not something to discuss. I changed the subject a little. "What do they do at the Alzheimer's Association? Is that something I should look into?"

"It isn't a medical facility. It's an information center, as I am led to believe. I imagine they have some good reading material. In time you may want to look into support services they can refer you to."

I construed that he hadn't looked them up and they hadn't looked him up. They probably sent him literature.

"How about the psychiatric facility at the hospital? Is that anything I should know about?"

Loughrand's style would never permit him to make a negative comment, but he was capable of pauses and slight adjustments of his eyes. "That's new. I don't know much about it. They work with children and adults who have emotional problems. They get into dementias, too." He was trying to recall exactly what they did do for a patient with a medical problem. From previous discussions I knew that Loughrand had never fully adjusted to psychiatry as a branch of medicine. I wasn't sure I had either.

"I hear you on the neurologist," I said. "I want to think a day or two before doing anything."

When I got home I called the Alzheimer's office. A warm-voiced woman said I could come right now or in the morning.

INA Krillman's office decoration consisted of shelves of books and pamphlets and a row of metal folding chairs arranged for a small meeting in front of a small desk that she dominated like an adult on a pony. She wore a street dress and hat, not a nurse's uniform, and as she came around the desk to shake hands and sit beside me on one of the metal chairs she tilted out of line in order to face me, I took her for a gray lady, one of the admirable women who keep organizations going, as Stella had been, but who are not the voices of authority. I thought I would get a pamphlet about the disease and another that advised caregivers to take care of themselves.

I was not prepared for a woman who had buried her mother after Alzheimer's, whose father was in his third year of it, and whose husband was down with emphysema. Not every one of the some two hundred Alzheimer's chapters around the country can be run by a woman like Ina because there isn't that much trouble going around to mold them. She put forward none of her life as a reference; it came out obliquely, enough so that I knew her knowledge was not out of a book.

She probed Stella's history out of me until she felt ready to say, "Let's say the diagnosis is confirmed and think ahead a little. Your wife will almost certainly start on tacrine. You know about tacrine, don't you?"

Dr. Loughrand and Carey Dingman had mentioned it. I had picked up an information sheet at the pharmacy. I understood it was all that was out there . . .

"Not quite. There are new drugs in clinical trials that probably would be glad to accept Mrs. Alterra. I am not recommending them or not, I'm just saying they're there. You will want to know about them. If not now, then perhaps in six months, because" — she made sure she had my attention — "tacrine is not for every patient. Many patients can't tolerate it at the effective dosage. You don't find out till you take it and the blood tests come back."

If not for every patient, how many were the lucky few? If there was no cure in any medication, what were the odds for us?

"It doesn't work in the sense of cure for anybody. Anybody who has Alzheimer's dies with it. Not of but with. It doesn't go away. My father had plateaus for a few months when the disease seemed to be at a standstill. There were the same plateaus before tacrine, after tacrine, and during tacrine. It is hard to say that a disease which has no predictable rate or sequence of progress can be said to be retarded by any intervention. We rely on researchers to see patterns in double-blind tests. They tell us that the drug has some effect in decreasing the rate of decline. You know about double-blind."

I knew the principle: a double-blind test compares the effect of a drug against that of a placebo in enough subjects to allow patterns of success and failure to emerge. Too many extraneous factors existed — family histories, prior illnesses, comparable lifestyles — and time was too short for satisfactory Alz double-blinds to be conducted. In the laboratory, tacrine had a positive effect on tissue. In the field, the side effects were significant but they could be monitored by blood tests and the drug discontinued if necessary.

Ina's mother hadn't been able to tolerate it at all, so one couldn't say it wouldn't have worked on her if she had been able to stay with it. "Her bilirubin shot right up. On the other hand, I had a woman — a nurse at that — tell me," and Ina wanted me to pay attention to this too, "that if her husband missed his forty milligrams for even one day she could tell. He died within a year after going on it. Even if it works, it doesn't work for very long. They don't prescribe it for more than a year or so. There you have it."

A few months was a few months. It could be years. In that time, a researcher might discover a silver bullet —

"You have to be mentally prepared that your wife — Stella? — won't be able to give it a good try because of its side effect. There is a large potential for liver damage. Patients on the drug are closely monitored. If the blood test shows liver damage, no more tacrine. There are other possible side effects but liver damage is the one we are most aware of." She saw it in a faint yellowing of her mother's complexion in the month between blood tests, before they saw it in the laboratory. Experimental drugs in clinical trials might be no more effective than tacrine but they did not attack the liver.

"Ina, if Stella were your mother, knowing what you know, what would you do tomorrow?"

She had no hesitation. "I would put her on Cognex through the first doctor who would write the prescription. A blood test would be a necessary preliminary. Stella already had that? Last week?"

The blood lab report was in Loughrand's hands yesterday. I had a copy. I asked for copies of lab reports. Sometimes there was something on them I could understand, like cholesterol readings or PSAs for prostate.

Ina said, "At the same time I would begin to plot to get her into a clinical trial at the first opportunity."

Plot seemed a strange word. Plotting meant establishing a relationship with Dr. Geerey. Geerey was a frequent consultant to a clinic that ran drug trials for major international pharmaceutical corporations. He also had a private practice in neurology. If Stella became his patient for Cognex and the medication did not succeed, she would be positioned with him to be recommended for the clinical trial of a promising experimental drug. There was a Japanese drug in trial. There was a Swiss drug. A double-blind, not practical for the diagnosis of Alzheimer's, has a place in differentiating the effect of one drug from another or from a placebo.

"If tacrine is so chancy, why wouldn't we go to the experimental drug right away?"

"I don't think you want to go into a trial unless you find out that Stella can't tolerate tacrine. In a trial she might not get any medication at all. A trial isn't a patient service, it's a research activity. She will enter a double-blind test for a period of weeks or months. She may get the drug. She may get the placebo. You want to be sure Stella is on a drug soon."

Carey Dingman had said that even a poor drug had a better chance to be effective in the disease's early stage. Ina endorsed Dingman.

"The patient has been ravaged long before Alzheimer's has been diagnosed — maybe months, maybe even years. I go by instinct. I believe the origins are way back. Not necessarily genetic, but long before they surface as Alzheimer's. Long before we imagine even in hindsight." Ina's instinct was that it was in her parents a long time ago. Not science, not provable, but way back. "When it surfaces it comes with a powerful rush. It's better to get started and stop if Alzheimer's is a false alarm," she dismissed it as unlikely, "than to lose time."

INA got us to Geerey the next day. He didn't do anything Loughrand hadn't done. He had read the blood lab report and talked to the technician at the radiology lab who told him there was nothing instructive on the CT scan. He asked Stella a few questions about her family, her drinking habits, gave her some drawing and memory tests, asked her to subtract seven from one hundred.

"Doctor," I said in an aside — Stella had become inattentive to asides, "we did sevens this morning. You may want to do another number." While sevens are the common test, they are not magic; other subtractions demonstrate the breakdown of function.

Geerey acknowledged the advice and went right on as if he hadn't heard. "Subtract for me seven from a hundred."

"Seven from a hundred?" Stella stalled, feeling for what was expected of her. She gave it a few seconds more and came up with a wrong number.

I FELT unfulfilled that Geerey had come to a conclusion as rapidly as Loughrand. From Neurology I had expected measurable science, which I knew of only as words: Sequential Multiple Analysis tests; folate, vitamin B12, and thyroid function analyses; a spinal tap. (If a spinal tap was simply a doctor's order for one more thing he wanted to know, I would have resisted vigorously on the irrational ground that I simply do not like the idea of spinal taps. They make me queasy. Like eating snails. I had heard also that they were painful. Pain was not something I would accept for Stella without a lot of justification.)

Not that I disbelieved Geerey, but I felt that Stella was owed something slower, more comprehensive. Mentally I was satisfied; emotionally I needed more. Therefore, during the week Dr. Geerey started Stella on Cognex we also went to the hospital's outpatient psychiatric facility and met Dr. Harrison, a cheerful, considerate man who gave the impression that his day belonged to us.

As far as Stella was concerned, it was just one more appointment to see if something could be done to improve her memory. Alan Harrison became Stella's mentor there for several half-day tests that, after the first morning, Stella characterized as she had Loughrand's: "dumb questions."

For some interviews we saw Harrison together, while he canvased our demeanors, testing our relationship and the reliability of our responses in the presence of each other. Psychiatrists have to suspect that all is not what meets the eye.

For a few minutes of each visit Stella was alone with him while I worked through *Good Housekeeping, People, Money,* and *Book Digest* in the waiting room and wondered what brought these other relatively young adults and children to psychiatry, a destination Stella and I had never before had. Eventually, she emerged with the day's clipboard sheaf of Harrison's multiple-choices to be completed before we went to lunch. "He talks to me like I'm a child," she said. "He asked me my birthday. When I told him, he said, 'That's *very* good.' I thought he would give me a lollipop. Doesn't everybody know her own *birthday?*"

In not many months, not everybody.

We sat side by side on office chairs, the clipboard in her lap. I declined Stella's attempts to enlist me in the choices. It would be like turning in somebody else's urine specimen. "It's your test, not mine."

She was not concentrating very well. The intensity of the experience tired her. I kept an eye out to be sure she did not drift off and lose track of the pages remaining. She tended to dwell on each *yes, no, often,* and *never* as if there were no other questions to go on to. She had lost the concept of pacing herself, the perception that disposing of 35, 37, and 46 in no more seconds than was necessary to circle Yes or No had a relationship to getting to 200 by closing time.

At a few questions I pointed out that she had circled both Yes and No. "You answered those questions the way your son might when he is in a challenging mood. Here you're allowed only one answer. Yes or No, which do you like?"

I also kept an eye out for unintended answers that might encourage the interrogator to suspect that whatever else was the matter with her, she was probably also on drugs and alcohol, was depressed, suicidal, and hated her father. One or another version of those questions kept coming up. Casual errors might be canceled by the weight of contrary evidence, but some might indelibly stain the examiner's subconscious so that at the end of the day *None of the above* would not prevail against one clue that Stella needed a fifth of sherry to get through the afternoon.

"Did you mean to say you drink more than four ounces of whiskey before dinner?" I showed her what four ounces would look like in a glass.

"Me?"

"It's your test. Do you want to tell Dr. Harrison that you take four drinks before dinner?"

"I don't usually drink anything before dinner."

"That's what to tell him. You don't want him to think you're an alcoholic. I'll erase the circle around 4. Put it around 0."

More telling, I thought, than her answers to any question and her leisurely progress from one to the next was her consistent failure to gauge the amount of space her writing took on a line. When she signed her name at the foot of each page, nothing could induce her to be aware of the limited space provided. Her signature marched overconfidently toward the margin, leaving room for only a cramped squiggle of the last few letters. On test questions that required more than Yes, No, or Choose, her sentences ran into margins. When I called it to her attention she huddled spidery words at the beginning of lines as she had for Dr. Loughrand.

I don't think Harrison had to get all those questions answered before he knew. Her compacted signature on the first page would have alerted him. Loughrand might not have had to go even as far as the sevens before he made the educated guess that Stella had Alzheimer's. He might have seen it in the way she signed her name in his secretary's log. Of course, nobody can act finally and irretrievably on such little evidence, but the compass needle surely swung.

ALz has only a downward course, with occasional plateaus for unpredictable weeks or months in which specific declines seem to be arrested while others continue downward. The best that could be expected of Stella's medication was that it slowed the rate of deterioration.

For researchers, such questions are answered by tests that forecast typical behavior of groups with and without medication. Quite a few individuals might not exhibit typical behavior. The course of the disease itself is erratic; the rate of decline varies from case to case, from symptom to symptom. Stella was an individual. For me, knowing the variety of symptoms and the apparently random sequence in which they occurred, the question was, What value did the medication have for Stella? It was never resolved. Instead, I acted on Pascal's principle: if faith entails no great loss, and the possible gain is substantial, why not act on it?

The immediate fact was the possibility of a good result. To get there, Stella needed to be at the effective forty-milligram level as quickly as possible. If that level was dangerous, blood tests would give warning. Proceeding from an opening minimum bid of ten milligrams, which almost every patient tolerated, the clinic stepped it up to twenty milligrams. If ten was so widely tolerated, why not begin at twenty?

Having begun at ten, why not salvo to thirty and retreat if necessary to twenty? I asked. This was war. In war, real generals were not bound by books written at leisure in academies. They overpowered the center. They attacked the flank. Their object was to be effective. My object was to get to the effective dose. Days now counted.

The clinic's case was that the patient's ability to assimilate the drug was progressive; small steps may have had minimum value, but they prepared the body to accept higher doses. Creeping fire, not salvo. In another month the blood lab signaled that Stella could move up to thirty milligrams. I pressed again to skip to forty and they responded again that protocol derived from experience and required the step advance to thirty.

Had I seen a glimmer of the disease's cessation I might have had less anxiety about the delay, but Stella had been slipping steadily since Loughrand's initial diagnosis. It was as if being recognized professionally as Alzheimer's had empowered it. Stella's speech was becoming terser. Her ability to shop, to manage the kitchen, to make social arrangements, to keep track of her calendar had diminished rapidly. Of her own volition she had given up driving.

I arranged with Grita Tomaz, a paragon of housekeepers who had come to us for a few hours a week for many years, to give us as much time as she could spare from her other commitments. I knew that her talents extended far beyond housekeeping; on days she did not come to us she went to a chronically ill housebound patient and to another who, although now in a nursing home, would not relinquish Grita who still came to read to her, exercise her, patiently urge her through meals.

In *Another Name for Madness*, Marion Roach's headlong memoir of her mother's life with Alzheimer's, she writes of a woman, long in the transient employment of the family, who became nurse and companion to the woman for whom she had kept house, and also became the patient's closest friend. I can say no less of Grita, who did everything a loving mother could do for Stella and who also became her closest friend. I mutter an exception under my breath, "Second to me," but I am not sure which of us was less dispensable.

We soon needed more days than Grita could give us and turned to home-care agencies. I respect the training and the commitment brought to this demanding work by women sent over from agencies, but nothing equals having the vocation. Grita, who had no certificate or even an hour of formal training, had an instinct for the right thing to do. She saw everything, overheard doctors and nurses, forgot nothing, and made tactful suggestions when the caregiver himself, her employer, did not do as well as she could for her patient.

Grita encouraged Stella to walk, to exercise, to look through old Christmas and birthday cards and photo albums, to crayon and watercolor the outlined scenes in drawing books. With her left hand she kept the house in order, did laundry, prepared meals, and stocked the freezer with casseroles and pastries. Apparently undisturbed emotionally by the changes in her life, Stella ceded all responsibilities, except that she occasionally looked into the kitchen to see what was going on.

Mindful of urgings by authorities that the caregiven be encouraged to participate in their historic roles, Grita or I — whichever was wearing the cook's hat for that meal — invited Stella to pour a cup of milk into the bake-mix, butter bread, set the table, push the first button of the blender. A kitchen has no production line; simple tasks are done in moments and there is no backlog of uncomplex undone work for someone whose skills are gone. There are only so many stones in lentils, so many rotting raspberries to be culled from a box, so many eggs to be beaten. Stella could not adjust flames, handle knives or boiling pots, take anything from the broiler or toaster oven, do anything electrical except push a blender or coffeemaker button or depress the toaster lever. Her interest quickly flagged.

AT the clinic, before we got through thirty milligrams, Stella's liver refused the test, reflecting an inability to "take up, process, and secrete bilirubin into the bile."

While I did not rejoice in the failure, I was mentally prepared to move to the clinical trial of the leading-edge drug that had whatever values were in tacrine, plus a very high probability that there would be no liver damage. But before Stella could be accepted in the trial her liver would have to regain its normal health. When they predicted the recovery would be rapid they were not talking days.

"Four weeks. Perhaps six."

I had expected that if tacrine failed we would move quickly to the new drug. No one had warned me otherwise. I began to think like cancer patients who go to Mexico for treatment with drugs not approved in the United States. My invaluable daughter-in-law at the hospital turned up literature on Dr. Chaovance Aroonsakul in Naperville, Illinois. Aroonsakul had specialties in neuro-gerontology and molecular biology and a practice based on her own research in 1984 and later work of Dr. Bengt-Ake Bengtsson, professor of endocrinology at Gotebord University in Sweden. Could anyone fail to be impressed? Stated simply, Bengtsson's theory was that inasmuch as Alzheimer's, like Parkinson's, resulted from neurodegeneration it could be treated with hormone replacement therapy as Parkinson's was.

Validating Aroonsakul, the FDA allowed the treatment, Medicare covered the office visits, and the IRS allowed the other costs on the medical line, subject to the same threshold deduction as other medical expenses. I noted with skepticism, however, that Aroonsakul supported her theory with only seven patient histories before creating the Alzheimer's and Parkinson's Disease Diagnostic and Treatment Center. While not averse to choosing a venturesome option, I was reluctant to gamble Stella's fate while the option of entering the new drug trial at a nearby clinic remained unexploited.

What riveted my attention was that Dr. Aroonsakul reported success in reversing — *reversing!* — Alzheimer's. At least I could make a phone call.

I spoke to an associate of Dr. Aroonsakul, by voice a sober man not given to extravagant statement. I detected no quackery.

Could he refer me to doctors in New York or Massachusetts who were committed to the therapy? No, we would have to come to Chicago. We would have to live there for an indefinite amount of time. Close monitoring of the patient was especially critical. But —

"Did you say your wife had to discontinue tacrine because it affected her liver? We would not be able to do anything for her until the bilirubin normalizes."

The Illinois clinic could begin doing its thing no sooner than the local clinic could begin doing its thing. For the time being at least, I put aside the possibility of moving to Illinois.

HERBAL remedies outside the medical mainstream were also available. To ensure that I considered natural healing and did not reject it out of hand as I had rejected their generation's music, our children saw to it that I read the underground literature of vitamins, minerals, and plants. Being a practiced agnostic in such things, I was as prepared to believe as to disbelieve. Lecithin, vitamin E, and ginkgo were recurrent words and recurrent labels in health food stores. Broccoli extract had advocates. These preparations were packaged by small companies that could not afford the expensive FDA routine. To avoid FDA challenge, claims on packages were circumspect. Not similarly disciplined, health store circulars carried testimonials from satisfied users at least as persuasive as the double-blind test tables of mainstream medicine.

I consulted three doctors, including the senior hepatologist at a teaching hospital, about all the alternatives. They concurred that in the presence of liver damage, no drug should be taken, whether of conventional provenance or promoted in astral sign pamphlets, and using any regime precluded using others. If Stella's liver again rejected a drug, how would we know which was the culprit if she took more than one at a time?

I had to choose the next therapy, and no matter which course I chose, Stella had to first wait one month — which became two months — and finally three horrendous months in which all drugs were suspended while her bilirubin number failed by tantalizingly decreasing margins to return to the norm and her capacities diminished remorselessly.

AFTER the liver hazard came the placebo. The trial in which Stella was enrolled had a narrow focus and the ratio of drug to placebo users was high — three drug users to one placebo user. I had hoped the clinic manager would be able to manipulate her supply to beat even those good odds and assure that Stella was on medication, but she couldn't do it; the packets were assembled elsewhere; the clinic staff knew no more than the patient what was in each packet. All that was done locally was match numbers. It was the trial's business to protect itself against plausible petitions like mine.

"I wouldn't worry if I were you," the manager said. "With three to one odds —"

She was wrong — if she were me she would worry. "Stella has been without effective medication all these months. Isn't there some way to be sure?" She regretted there was none. However, the trial would be over in two months. After that, Stella would be eligible to enter an observation trial: all drug, no placebo. Stella would then get the drug that was not available for prescription for as long as she tolerated it — a year or more.

I didn't intend to give Stella any placebos. When we came home from the clinic, I opened a capsule in the packet of a month's supply and found a white powder. I put a pinch on my tongue and tasted nothing — not bitter, not sweet, not starch, not sugar — the closest texture and taste was finely ground sawdust. I spooned it into a plastic bag and took it to the hospital lab. I asked if they could do a test that would tell me if it was a drug — any kind of drug — or a harmless substance.

The attendant inquired in a back room and reported. "We don't do any testing here. We send our work to a lab in Boston." He gave me the name and number from his phone chart. The name was of a drug company so huge that I foresaw miles of paperwork and days of waiting for a report. I telephoned and told them what I had told the hospital and got a prompt answer. "We don't do testing for private individuals."

Did they know anybody who did?

They did not. The blinkered disinterest of well-placed people about the fringes of their own daily work must create many openings for others to better themselves. If I worked for a lab I would know the name of every other lab on the scene and what it did. I can't tell you specifically what good that would do me, but I do have a romantic conviction that to know is better than not to know. I thought of the lab I should have thought of first — the police lab. The police must be able to test quickly for street drugs: marijuana, amphetimines, cocaine. It's a small town; you walk in and see the right people. I handed the desk sergeant the plastic envelope and put to him the question I had asked the hospital.

"We don't have much of a laboratory. We test only for controlled substances."

"That would be fine. I don't want to know what it is. All I want to know is if it's anything at all or nothing. Can you do that?"

"We might be able to do that. Come back in the morning."

In the morning he handed me an official envelope with a tag stating that no controlled substance had been found. "Your grandchildren visiting?" he asked with polite suspicion.

"That's close enough," I said.

"If we had found anything we might have had to ask you some questions."

I went to the clinic manager's office.

"My wife seems to be on a placebo. I'm sorry, we can't take that. We've lost too much time."

"How do you know what it is?"

"Assume I know. I'm going to have to take Stella off your program." I exaggerated a little: "We can get into a trial in Boston beginning tomorrow with better odds. It may not be as good a drug but it won't be a placebo. I'm sorry but I can't let Stella go any longer without medication."

"I was going to call you," she said. "We had somebody drop out of an observation program. Stella can begin our program tomorrow." She smiled companionably. "How does that sound?"

The next day when we got the new packet I opened a capsule and put my tongue to the powder. It would enhance my ego to say at this point that my detective talent was confirmed; that the powder was mordantly bitter and that for the first time I felt sure Stella was getting the best available medicine. The fact is this powder was as bland as the other. The texture was somewhat coarser, a difference that may have been in my imagination.

I returned to the clinic and told the manager, "I need to be reassured that this is not a placebo."

Those within a system know that their duty is to the system, not to the public. Nevertheless, we always hope that in the instant case, different standards prevail. I looked her in the eye when I said I needed reassurance, and I accepted her direct gaze when she replied, "It's the real McCoy."

In the interim after Loughrand's diagnosis and before Stella entered clinical trial of the Swiss drug Sandoz ENA 713 her decline was more marked than at any time since. She had been without even theoretically effective medication for seven months before going on 713. Add the earliest months in which Alz had probably been active without being identified and Stella had been very long — I don't want to think how long; maybe more than a year — without meaningful medical care. And yet, I had proceeded more resourcefully than most caregivers might have.

While the dosages of the new drug advanced in scheduled increments, Stella's disorientations became more frequent, her language became shorthand, walking strength deteriorated so that she was secure only with an escorting arm or a cane. I have rarely felt as entirely helpless in my life as I did then. Stella was slipping out of my hands. Her name no longer sprawled into the margin of documents or huddled like an exercise in writing on the head of a pin; her signature became mine, under durable power of attorney.

I credit Sandoz ENA 713 for the relatively gentle slope of her subsequent decline, especially in intellection and social skills. Her physical disabilities — walking, feeding, toileting, writing — continued to slide, but less precipitously. The whole mood of deterioration changed from swift decline to moderation. Whether this was cause and effect or merely co-incidental can be argued, but not to me. I have continued to feel that 713 slowed the inexorable tide.

Now and then I touch my tongue to ENA 713; it always tastes like sawdust. Surely, I tell myself, even the most malign system would not have been giving Stella a useless powder all this time. I continue to believe that at least that one time I made the right choice for Stella.

4

GIVING UP THE KEYS

A<small>T THE</small> V<small>ILLAGE</small> N<small>URSING</small> and Retirement Residence small groups of seniors (not necessarily with Alzheimer's but who had some impairment or were merely aged) met one or two days a week to do crafts, discuss the headlines, exercise, visit gardens and galleries.

I thought the Residence senior group might be for Stella, although in her best years she had not been much of a joiner.

She had membership cards and paid dues to a dozen — perhaps dozens — of organizations appropriate to her means and interests, everything from the Symphony Society to Common Cause, but she seldom went to meetings she could avoid. I thought she might change. At the time, Stella had begun taking tacrine but not yet found out that her liver would not accept it. I don't remember what ruse I used to induce her to ride over to the Village Residence with me to see what went on.

The receptionist led us to a room in which a dozen seniors and two or three staff members were in the midst of morning activities. They were playing bingo. Apparently they had had a party; several were wearing clown hats. Posters of crayoned stick figures and simple landscapes were hung around the room. I didn't have to look at Stella's face to see her nose twitch. It wouldn't seem to her to be an adult environment. The woman in charge asked us if we would like to sit in for a while. Stella signaled me that she was ready to leave. I explained to the woman that we wanted only to take a look at the facility, thanked her, and we left.

I needed to regroup. I asked Ina at the Alzheimer's Association office for guidance. She said, "Village Residence? That's a day care. I think you're looking for support groups." I didn't know there was a difference. Ina explained that day care was for people functioning at a lesser level of competence than Stella and not at all for caregivers. "We have something going here in the chapter that might be for both you and Stella."

They had separate caregiver and caregiven groups that met for an hour every other week. Ina referred to the two groups as caregivers and spouses, which they were most often, but sometimes they were siblings or parent and child. In one room, caregivers compared experiences and resources and exchanged advice. On the other side of the wall, spouses talked about anything that came up — their favorite foods and TV programs, what they liked and didn't like about what went on at home. They talked about places they had visited and their children.

"Sometimes they talk about their husbands," Ina said. "But you will never know what they say. It is held within the group."

I did not expect Stella to be enthused. She might find it interesting, might meet people she liked. Sessions lasted only an hour. I would be in the adjoining room with the caregivers. If it didn't work out, all she had to do was tell me at the end of the hour and we would not return.

Glancing around the spouses' meeting room I had an impression of an ordinary group of women gathered to hear a talk at the library, women not even especially elderly for our part of the world, where there were many retirees. To enhance fellowship, the rule of admission was that they must be in the early stage, not the advanced; the first year into Alzheimer's (maybe the second, it's always hard to say how long the damn thing went on before the diagnosis). Years and tests were not what counted, the demeanor of early Alz was looked for.

Stella was put off by a woman I later knew as Alma, whose husband Dan Boudreau I would meet on the other side of the wall. Alma's speech and somber manner implied mental impairment. "That woman's not all right," Stella muttered to me. I thought bleakly of Groucho Marx who would not join a club that would have him as a member. A woman we had met a few years ago recognized Stella and greeted her.

"See you later, Stell. I'll be in the next room," I said.

I left her with Lenore, the meeting facilitator sent in by the chapter, and joined the assembling caregivers next door.

I DID not need to be entertained or have my time more occupied than it was, nor did I feel the social need to be among my spousal peers. I joined to hear the experiences of other caregivers, and in trade for theirs I expected to disclose some of mine. A pleasant surprise — the facilitator on our side of the wall was Ina. At the opening go-round to introduce ourselves, she led to loosen us up: "My father has Alzheimer's, sixth year." Three times as long as any of us had been with it. Mother and father, both Alzheimer's. Her husband, emphysemic. Ina expected God's chillun to have troubles, among them the care of an invalid. When the phone rang after a day in which Ina had heard nothing but hard stories it may have been her son who never made it and could use a few dollars; it could be her daughter who lived an indefinite life.

In the several times we had spoken I had come to think of Ina as the figurehead of a clipper ship, veteran of long voyages in all weather who had earned time for a little coastal carrying, but she went where the orders sent her; not for the walking around money the Alz office afforded but because it was something she did well on a schedule she could handle. Inside her was the armature of a Sargent matron: busty, narrow-waisted, haunchy. She and her husband used to dance a lot. She remembered ballrooms and the names of bands that played Berlin and Porter and Arlen. "Oh I did like to dance," Ina said. I thought she probably still did. When she said it her face became vivacious, as the faces of older women often do when they remember dancing.

I guessed I was the oldest in the group. It would have been generous to call the youngest man late middle-aged. The only woman, though, was in her forties. Dorothy was married to the older man in the other room.

It didn't follow necessarily that the cadre next door was our mirror image, six women, one man: women could be caring for mothers, men for brothers. At other times women predominated on both sides of the wall. Women are still the caretakers of children and parents, they outlive us and are therefore more often invaded by old age's hallmark disease. The groups met every second week for an hour, in cycles of six meetings. New people could join at any time; there wasn't an organized curriculum. Every meeting was what the members wanted it to be. Some couples came for a few meetings but left because of schedule conflicts, or it became a reach to drive an hour to get to a group that met for an hour. Some of those with Alzheimer's discovered after a session or two that they didn't want to be with depressed people or people who talked about themselves all the time or who fell asleep. When they opted out, the spouses went too.

Usually departures were because over weeks or months some spouses descended too far into the jungle of the disease and the caregiver withdrew them, or the maestra Lenore saw that a profoundly disoriented person created problems of behavior and image — the image that less-afflicted members of the group and their caregivers had of themselves. Again the Groucho Marx syndrome. As time passed, some participated with vigorous irrationality. Some ceased to be responsive to the environment; they dozed. Lenore would take the caregiver aside and tactfully make it known that perhaps it was not a good idea to sign up for the next three months.

In the caregivers' group, therefore, were old hands whose spouses had endured. They brought to the table not only their own experiences but the remembered experiences of others. I came to the group as one of the new boys and became an old hand when Stella said she enjoyed it and wanted to stay with it another term. In some ways she had fallen below Lenore's standard of eligibility, but as she had a gift of social presence she seemed less afflicted than she was.

In a half year, about twenty pairings joined, departed, stayed. A law of averages must have operated to keep us at seven pairs, plus or minus a pair or two. No phenomenon is more remarkable than the laws of averages; not gravity, not space.

TODAY we are trading experiences about spouses giving up driver's licenses. Horton says with some satisfaction that his wife still drives. He is a man of dominant personality, vice president of a large corporation before he retired with the financial benefits of office.

"Your wife is still *driving?*" Dan blurts. He usually speaks with the circumspection of a salesman dealing with people who write orders. That Horton's wife drives catches him off balance; he has seen Marie in the hall and on the way to the parking lot. She seems to be as unfocused as Alma and Alma doesn't drive; there is an injustice. "You let her drive a *car?*"

Some of us here live by monthly checks and since Alz began have been going down the financial drain. Dan is on the low end. He kept working after passing his expected retirement age, and took up similar work elsewhere. He goes from store to store selling specialty foods, filling racks, delivering emergency orders that won't wait for the Thursday truck, discouraging delinquent payments without losing the account. His hair has drawn away from the patch it occupied when his hairpiece was new and the piece is now something a monk or a religious Jew could wear in a pinch. He has a friendly, joke-telling way and impresses me as a man who always thought he was on the verge of doing better; he is in it now for the calls he has time to spare from caring for his wife. Most days he leaves her from nine to three to do the best she can for herself.

Horton and Marie are well off although not chauffeur-driven, which may be their choice; in Horton is a lot of New England's wintry frugality that does not show its hand. He and Marie have a housekeeper, and a man comes to garden and do minor carpentry. Last Fourth of July the support group pic-nicked at his house on a few acres of meadow at the bend of a river. It had been their summer place. On a table was a photo of a younger Horton and Marie at the door of a more vice-presidential kind of house with pillars.

Horton has another, rarer kind of wealth for a man whose wife has early stage Alzheimer's: several able and willing daughters settled within easy reach. Dan Boudreau's children and mine, Kevin's and Dorothy's may be equally gifted but they are in California or Canada or Maryland. Sometimes a daughter comes with Horton to see her parents' Alz support group for herself.

Kitty is the third Horton daughter we have met. She has her father's way in groups, is undoubtedly chairperson of committees, and is not bashful in the presence of seniors. The idea of Mom's foot on the gas pedal of a four-door Oldsmobile scares her. "Scares the heck out of me." There have been dis-cussions about this at home. She speaks to us as a way of speaking to her father. She may have come to find allies.

"Mom drives adequately but she was never really a great driver. Her reactions now are slower. I worry about her at an intersection where a lot is going on, don't you, Dad?"

Horton is not used to criticism from the bottom up. At home he may say, "I'm not going to take the car away from your mother until she is ready," and return to his newspaper. Here he must make a public defense. His eyes and jaw withdraw the endorsement they have given his executive smile.

"Marie likes to drive. It gives her the feeling that she is in control of an important part of her life. When she's unsure about driving — on account of the weather or because we're going a distance — she herself suggests that somebody else take the wheel. It's only a couple of blocks to the market and about the same to church. She drives carefully."

"It takes only a second of inattention and something happens you can never take back," Kitty says.

Horton does not accept that as a serious argument. "It can happen to any of us. We won't deny your mother the pleasure while she can enjoy it."

Daughters may then have to be quiet but the rest of us are free to offer second opinions. Dan has regained his composure. He asks genially, "Are you waiting for an accident?"

STRANGERS though we may be, knowledge of what it is to live with Alzheimer's in the house tends to make us easy with each other. It is different here from with friends who ask, "How are things going?" and wait a little longer for an answer than from "Hello, how are you?"

"I'm glad you asked" is not a good answer to friends; we don't want to take advantage of courteous questions. The situation is marginally uncomfortable, like first words to the bereaved. A given of Alz is that things are no better than yesterday; concern is sufficiently acquitted in the asking. "Level" is a good answer.

Do you really want to know — do I really want to tell you? — that Stella pulled the bedroom window shades off their brackets, some off their rollers? She must have been puzzled when the first one kept coming until it fell around her and she went on to the next window, sensing wrong, trying to get to a place where the process would end. She didn't call for help. I thought she acted strangely when she came from the bedroom hall, as if she had something to say but didn't have the words.

Stella had just been obliged to go off her first medication and was waiting for her liver to clean up before going into the clinical trial. Her slide seemed to be accelerating. She came into the sitting room and simply stood, looking in a way familiar to me when she was puzzled about what to do next. "Stell, is there something I can do for you?"

It wasn't the best way to ask; I had begun to learn that choosing is something a person with Alzheimer's doesn't do well, especially abstract choosing. A choice between a baked apple and a brownie on the table can be made; between only the words that represent them, choice is difficult but possible. To make an unprompted choice, however, in a world of possibilities — *anything* I can do for you — without even multiple-choice answers to select from, may be too much.

Every case is a different cluster of lost faculties, but difficulty in making choices is as common as symptoms get. And if she says "No" she may mean yes. If Stella says "Yes" she may be merely acknowledging the subject, not expressing a preference. If she says "Yes" and does not go on to say what it is she wants me to do, she may have forgotten what she wants. The open-ended question establishes only that we are in question-and-answer mode. It means Are you ready? Here comes the question: "Would you like a glass of orange juice?" She said, "I would like that."

She then asked if she could sit in that chair, which is the chair she always sits in facing the TV. My wife of more than fifty anniversaries asking humbly where she may sit may seem trivial to you; not to me. I hate the idea that one human being, having come to sufficient maturity, feels obliged to ask another's permission to sit on a certain chair in her own home. I hate the idea that any person — I — is seen to be so privileged as to make such decisions. May my wife sit in her own chair? In her own home? In our marriage we had had conflicts of will, but decisions had not been imposed or conceded to shouting or unexplained yesses and nos. And yet I was asked for permission. I tried to give the decision back to her. "It's your house — sit wherever you want to." She may not have meant to ask permission. It was a way of saying the available options of chairs and sofas bewildered her at the moment, in whatever complex of ideas and emotions she was dealing with. She wanted guidance. "Why don't you sit here?" I pointed to the chair. It helps to gesture.

She sat. I got the orange juice. While I was up I thought to see if anything in the bedroom had caused her to look so bemused when she came from the hall. The bedroom was a surf of window shades. They lay across beds and dressers and spilled to the floor.

My peers in the support group understood when I said that I then behaved like an idiot. I came back to her shouting, demanding to know what she thought she was doing, ordered her to leave the shades alone, never do it again. Gaining imperial stature from her bewilderment, her failure to reply, I went on to explain with bitten anger how window shades operate, what must be done if rollers don't catch and so on, knowing while I carried on that this was an idiotic, monstrous, primitive way to behave. Being obliged to choose already had her in irons; adding noise, speaking rapidly, showing anger massively confused her. She did not see what was expected of her and did not know where to hide from the challenge. Her face disintegrated from bewilderment to panic while I tried to lower the heat without giving up my rational right to be angry; until she cried, the first time in years I had known her to cry. I put my arms around her and we made it up.

I could tell that to the caregivers. They too had behaved like idiots and been ashamed. They knew not only from books that an Alzheimer patient simply does not know how it happened, has lost the concept of one-thing-leads-to-another for hundreds of habitual acts. They too have shouted, employing the corrective power of noise because it is one of the ways we educate children to what is serious. Our lifelong habit of explaining; our belief that education happens as a result of telling, showing, and shouting; the very concept of educating this other person, all this has to be purged from the mind and habit of the caregiver.

An essence of Alz, to add to early loss of memory, is that the afflicted can no longer learn. In my experience it is not quite true, but it is true enough to be a rule of expectation: Do not give someone with Alzheimer's an instruction about how something is done with any expectation that it will then be remembered and done that way. Almost certainly, the instruction will be immediately forgotten. If there is no longer the possibility of education, will the window shades come down again? They may, but it is unlikely that the several accidents required to achieve the final calamity will again conspire: being alone, the shades within wavering reach, the concept of what a shade is for, the concept of how it is controlled, the perception that she is the one to do it.

The caregiver does his part by rearranging the furniture and repeating at the right time every evening that he does windows. The mantra may or may not have effect. If the shades come down again, the caregiver will shrug and let it go as one of those things. It will not be that he represses anger; in time he will have divested himself of anger.

Many odd acts like the riot with the window shades are never repeated. She was utterly confused — once — about how to get into a car beside the driver. After struggling with how to begin, she entered by crossing her right leg over the left. Her right foot anchored in the well in front of the seat required her to face backward to bring in the rest of herself. She had to be untangled. After that she sometimes stuttered between left and right but always decided correctly to get into a car left foot first.

One more turn with the window shades: Several days passed before I restapled the shades to the rollers and got up on a chair to rehang the first one. It didn't fit. The wooden roller had mysteriously shrunk. Anybody who has ever hung a window shade knows the phenomenon. It had become an eighth of an inch too short to seat in the brackets that had received it for ten years. The pin in one end and the tab of the spring device in the other merely rested on the brackets; a sideways jog or drift would unseat the whole contraption.

A slightly off-center tug and it would come down.

I tested the other rollers. The seats were a little firmer, but only a little. An off-center tug would bring them down. So. Very little of the disaster could be laid to her. Perhaps only the going on and on.

Consumed by guilt, I went to her and again apologized. I explained. She had no idea what I was talking about. She knew window shades and had a slight recall of them falling to the floor or being on the floor, or perhaps she agreed to what I was saying mostly to please me. But essentially it was all gone from her memory.

In the beginning she had lost only nouns and episodes of long-term memory; the warned-of loss of recent memories soon followed. Then memories of how to make sentences, the sequence of days, how to put one foot in front of the other, intellection — everything crumbles, as in movies of rivers in flood, breaking through dikes, overrunning them, inundating the low ground except for random hummocks of refuge, and rising inexorably toward the once-safe house.

I can't very well tell the window shade anecdote to friends. They are her friends too and they may have an edge of feeling that I am demeaning her. I should not volunteer disclosures to which she is helpless to put her own coloration. It distances me, as if I am withdrawing some of my stake in her. Instead of protecting her inadequacies I am exposing them. It violates the privacy of a marriage.

What I cannot tell my friends whom I know well I can tell my Alz group, people I don't know outside the meeting room. If it is the first time these chance acquaintances have heard of window shades coming down, they know something like it: a lamp put in the trash, an empty milk carton in the oven, results disconnected from intentions.

They know choices should be limited to this or that — and maybe even that overloads the circuit, the fuse blows and no light goes on. They know dependency and docility, and the opposite: the irrational resistance and rage of the sentient human core trying to make itself known in the unfamiliar shadow.

WE bring our footnotes of disaster to the group, sometimes to solicit guidance from someone who has been there, sometimes to give it, sometimes simply to share frustrations. They understand dependency, that Stella asks for permission to sit on a chair in her own home, and the other face of dependency: defiance of common sense, the assertion of person with whatever tool is at hand. Dorothy says Ray sometimes refuses to take off his glasses before stepping into the shower. She waits a few seconds, introduces an intervening distraction — here is your washcloth — and when she comes back to the glasses he allows her to lift them off without objection.

I told them that two days after the disaster Stella had forgotten the shades. Forgetfulness could be a blessing.

Dan said, "My wife would have blamed me for pulling down the shades. She would tell everybody that I pulled down the shades and blamed it on her. I'd never hear the end of it." Every person with Alzheimer's is different.

In the group before I joined it was a father, caregiver for a daughter in her early forties, among the youngest patients known to anybody around here. I know about this pair only as others speak of them. I can't think about a daughter in Alz, literally can't think about it. Like counting down from a thousand to get to sleep, my mind won't dwell on being around to spoon-feed a daughter breakfast cereal and unbind her head from the sleevehole of a sweater, to stand by while she toilets (for a half dozen reasons, some of which may not occur to you: Will the whole roll unwind while she tries to snap off a few sheets? Will she forget to drop her panties before she sits?). I'm not a prayer, but when I heard about the daughter, I muttered, "God of Job, save this scourge for the old."

I can't explain how I defend absolutely my right to be Stella's caregiver but couldn't handle my daughter were she in her mother's place. André Dubus wrote a story about a young woman who kills a man in a highway accident, leaves the scene more in bewilderment than with criminal intent, and comes home to her father for comfort and refuge. Her father wrestles with the problem of duty: Shall he persuade her to turn herself in? Shall he do it for her? In the end he absolves himself from the obligation, reasoning that the Lord allowed his son to be crucified but it is unthinkable that he would have stood aside while it happened to a daughter. Dubus's story casts a slant light on the peculiar relationship of fathers and daughters. I could take care of my son as I have his mother.

Today Ina hears the unproductive bicker developing between Dan and Horton. She enlarges the question. "How many of you have spouses who drive?"

Dorothy, new to the group and younger than the rest, bids with a discreet sign, as if it's a New York auction. She has a long, erect neck; hair hedges her face narrowly and bells out like an Egyptian queen's. The trace of a wound is on her upper lip, possibly a childhood operation for harelip. Her manner is observant, not because queens don't speak first but because if you are not much over forty, living in a problem of unimaginable complexity and duration, you touch before you grasp. They married when she was eighteen, he thirty-two. Compared to boys she knew, Ray must have seemed solid, mature. After our meetings, when the door opens and the spouses come out of the adjoining room, the sun-bronzed slow-moving man with the kindly eyes is Dorothy's. It is rare for a man in his middle fifties to have Alzheimer's. He waits to be last through the door. It may be out of courtesy. It may be that he is slowest to find the direction and the purpose.

The presence of Horton's daughter, more her peer than we are, may have encouraged Dorothy to respond without being asked directly. "Ray drives. He is early Alzheimer's."

All our spouses are "early Alzheimers." None of us knows "late" or "intermediate" or "profound" Alzheimer's, except in literature or as we see it terminally in nursing environments. No doctor tells us when we cross a threshold and we are now *here*. They simply stop saying "early." After the first diagnosis of "early" or "stage I," Alzheimer's is what it is.

The symptoms of one early compared to another, the rates of change, and the kinds of disability and the random sequences in which they appear are so radically different that we all wonder if it is truly one disease. All the symptoms may gather to a common feeble end; in the meantime the order, the intensity, the number of years the course runs are unknown until they happen. *Merck* says: "No predictable stages or patterns can be discerned ... but cognitive decline is inevitable." I know of people with Alzheimer's in their eighth diagnosed year, still driving. Stella was still in her first when she gave up the keys. Life is unfair. Ina throws the switch toward me. "How did you get Stella to do that?"

Many people around town were, in my opinion, far less qualified than Stella to drive. They came stiff-armed out of their driveways, looking neither right nor left, went along relentlessly at ten miles an hour less than the allowed speed, veered for birds as for erupting volcanoes, and crashed intersections like unpiloted locomotives that had slipped the brake and were headed out of the yard until in their own good time they arrived at the post office plaza and straddled two parking spaces like owners of RVs and luxury sedans with delicate fenders.

Compared with them, Stella could have taught driver's education; but only by comparison.

I no longer rehearsed life-saving maneuvers from the passenger seat. I drove. I found reasons to assume her stops at the market and the dry cleaner's and save her the trips. On the few occasions she drove out alone I fidgeted until she was safely home again, but she had a license. I rehearsed scenarios to get it away from her. I could ask Dr. Loughrand to tell her to give it up. I could talk to the chief of police, he might tell her that a random list of drivers of certain ages was being called in as a spot-check, nothing personal, and lo and behold! she would be found wanting. I could take it up with the licensing registry and the insurance company. Knowing what I knew, they would want her off the road. They wanted a lot of people off the road but it had to be handled gingerly; as broad policy it was politically impossible to take on a constituency of the elderly and their families who thought they drove well enough, considering.

The way it happened I could not have foreseen. Leaving the market parking lot after shopping —

Shopping! A year before Stella was still driving to the market, shopping independently, writing checks, counting change, planning menus, managing the kitchen. A half year later she had lost all those skills and many more: Getting both legs and both arms in the correct holes of underpants/ sleeves/slacks, sometimes a hopeless tangle of inside-out, wrong side front, upside-down; let's begin again. That much gone! But still, a year later, so many undefiled islands of intelligence. She asked for the evening news programs and the Sunday morning talk shows. She asked for a Villa-Lobos tape. She knew family well and close friends — still does — and wanted to walk the uneven ground to garden places she treasured: a cove of ladies-slippers, a flush of azaleas in the midst of hemlocks. She got jokes fast: we're supposed to master a language that says quiet *down* but shut *up?* They don't have to be very good jokes. They used to have to be better.)

— she turned right instead of left, two miles from home, and went on and on the wrong way, through other towns, on sometimes familiar roads but landmarks were in the wrong places. Not just a half mile lost as the time before, but off the screen for two hours while police, state troopers, and I looked for her. I found her passing a post office, coming toward home from the wrong direction. She had passed within a few hundred yards of the homes of friends and gone by stores with telephones where she could have made a call, driving a great circle — all but the last mile that would have taken her back again to the market — beginning on the north shore, returning from the south. Bemused but composed, she might have gone on until the gas ran out.

"I don't know what I did. I was lost. I couldn't seem to get straightened out. I don't think I should drive anymore."

She did not have to say it twice. I turned in her license and gave her car to a good cause. Any time she should be some place I get her there or see that somebody else does. Only once has she mentioned that she might want to drive again. I heard her and we went on to other subjects. It is no longer rude not to take up any conversation she offers. Wait till she asks again. If she doesn't insist, let it lie. It went from her mind.

"You had it easy," Dan said. Hearing how the others struggled with the problem, I agreed.

Another point was raised to Horton. "It isn't only the damage she might do to herself. What about the risk to others?"

His daughter said, "You would never forgive yourself something like that. Her doctor said it might be time for Mom to give up her license."

Horton says, "He said we should think about it. It's premature. We'll play it by ear. If the time comes I don't think Mom will be hard to convince."

Ina said, "Insurance might be something to think about. If there's an accident and the insurance company gets wind of the fact that her doctor said she shouldn't drive — they might not cover."

Dan said, "Nobody is rich enough to pay for an uncovered accident. It could be millions of dollars. If it's a baby with all her life still ahead, it could be a lot of millions."

"I'm aware of that," Horton said. Like Kitty, he was beginning to find it scary. Whether it was the time bomb moving into a downtown intersection or the multimillion dollar jury award that had his attention, the subject was open.

Boudreau asked a question from his own life: "What if as soon as she gets home after you've taken her somewhere she wants to go out again? Always on the go. What's the strategy?"

Ina said, "Sometimes you have to say, 'Sure, in an hour.' Put it off. Try not to prolong the discussion. Change the subject. Change it to something for her. Would she like to have a Coke? Is there something on TV she might like? Act as if the subject of the car is dead for now and go on to something else. As a last resort you can always excuse yourself to go to the bathroom."

I said that from my experience I thought she would forget it in a few minutes.

Boudreau said from his experience, "You think."

Every individual history is different.

THEY called each other Boudreau and Lady. Lady was at Penneman Pond, a 1920s estate that would be a Catholic seminary or a corporate retreat if it had not become a retirement/nursing home. Boudreau lived nearby. We were talking costs one morning in the Alz group and Boudreau gave us figures he had worked up. It cost fifty thousand dollars a year to keep Lady at Penneman. If he went down one day as he would have to expect, the cost would double. For the two of them, Penneman's room, board, social services, nursing and housekeeping services, and programs would cost one hundred thousand dollars a year and it was going up, not quite as fast as college tuition, but fast enough. A hundred thousand dollars was the income from a million and a half dollars in u.s. bonds if you had them. You needed a little more to cover extravagances like hair cuts and maintenance of the eight-year-old Plymouth registered in a nephew's name and parked in the residence lot. A disarming man, Boudreau often talked as if he had no secrets, he told you anything you asked and much that you didn't. He seemed to have nothing to cover, no appearances to keep up.

"If you're going to keep your principal intact you need another two or three hundred thousand to generate the income to pay the federal tax," Horton said, as if reminding a junior that he had not done his homework. "You have income, you have tax."

Dan, who did all his homework while trying to talk himself out of insomnia, said, "And you need a little something for the tax on the income for the tax, and a little something more for the income for the tax on the tax. I stopped figuring. I don't pay it anyhow. Medicaid pays it. You either have a million or two or poverty enough to suit Medicaid. Anything in-between and you can't afford it, it will eat the securities you planned to leave to put your grandchildren through college."

A lawyer can tell you how to dispose of assets while keeping them. He may not tell you directly, he may poke at it with a stick as if it were roadkill, but you can see what he is doing. A third option is to put aside enough to pay the nursing home bills for a few months until you run out of money, which is what Boudreau had done for Lady. If you had a room, Medicaid then maintained you as before. If you didn't already have a room, it might not be easy to find a Medicaid room. "The government won't do business with you until you run out of money."

Lady didn't know Boudreau as her husband. She thought he was her husband's cousin. She thought he was her chauffeur. She didn't want him in her room. During the day she roamed Penneman, talking to herself or to anybody who overheard: that man is in my room again. She told the head nurse that Boudreau would not take orders. She would fire the son of a bitch but there was a law against firing people.

When we saw her in the hall, Lady had a worn, sleepless, angry look. When Boudreau approached she looked past him. If he tried to lead her she brushed him off; he was a panhandler she had rejected and never wanted to hear from again.

Boudreau reported this from time to time with a wry smile. It's the way things were. It was up to God.

It must have been extraordinarily hard to come all that way, to fulfill all his duties and not be loved at all, not even be tolerated, not at least be remembered as a man who was once loved. Worse: maybe he was never loved and that was all Lady remembered; she didn't remember pretending something else. Maybe Boudreau knew that — all the more was his heroism. If you were brash enough to ask, he might have said, "Yes, I guess that's how it was."

But maybe he would have said, "We were once lovers like everybody has a chance at."

I could believe that to Boudreau the order of his life had merely been reversed. Instead of redemption coming late it had come early and it had to last. It could seem to Boudreau that many had it worse.

I asked Ina if she knew others as sainted as Boudreau. "Only somewhat. I know another breed —"

She told me of a man who knew about Alz and concluded that his wife had it before she knew. He told her a conventional story, that he thought his life was getting away from him, that he wanted to start out again alone. If she would think about it, it might be good for her, too. Her immediate reaction might be anger, but she should think about it. He wanted to be fair. He would leave her the house and as much income as he could afford. She should regard it as a favor that he acted decisively so she didn't have to. She too would have another chance. Surely there was something better than living the only life they had in a stale marriage?

"I know what she said," I guessed.

"Right. She said he was a son of a bitch, the same thing Lady calls Boudreau. In a year she was diagnosed with Alzheimer's. Her son cared for her for many years before she went to a nursing home. Her husband lived on the West Coast and never saw her again."

ON the spouse side of the wall, Lenore throws out a question to get conversation going: Does anybody here drink cocoa for breakfast? How about you, Marie? Is it cocoa? Is it coffee? It's tea in your house? From here they may go on to what they like to eat, what they don't like, what they ate as children, is soup better in a cup or a bowl, do they watch TV when they eat, what does the caregiver do while they eat, do they like the caregiver to cut foods to bite-size, do they like big spoons or teaspoons.

Lenore brings up the daily news: Did anyone see on TV the rice being distributed in Somalia? The conversation turns solemn: Sometimes I don't feel wanted in my home. The maestra reminded them again that nothing said here should go outside the walls. It was a pledge for herself, for she wanted this to be a place where they could let it all out without a daughter or a husband or a doctor looking over their shoulders.

In practice, Lenore's theory did not work perfectly. They might not remember the pledge; Stella told me what she usually would after a visit anywhere; although, more likely, she forgot what it was she wasn't supposed to talk about.

She was still bothered by those she thought did not socialize in an expected way. She had always reached out to every kind of human misfortune, now she stiffened toward those who were markedly depressed or sad, as if her nerves of empathy were silting up like her nerves of memory. "They live all bad news" she said. "I never feel —" with a gesture that meant "like that" to finish the sentence.

I didn't know how it happened that she saw nothing of herself but her age in the others, or how in the silent hours of reverie at home she did not fall into patches of desolation, but I knew her as well as any person knows another and I am sure that any dark mood she may have had lasted no more than moments.

WE were in the hall after our hour ended, waiting for the door of the spouses' room to open. One of us said Ina was entitled to a month in the best seaside hotel on Cape Cod. The impossibility of a month amused her. Her church had women who did respite care. Respite was an afternoon, a weekend. A month?

She smiled generously. "Lend me an old Visa you aren't using."

The door of the spouses' room opened: another group that looked much like any group of women getting off the senior bus at the museum. Stella seemed very tired. I held her hand and asked how the meeting had been, while Lenore took Ina aside and said a word to her. In a moment Ina caught my eye.

"Lenore thinks it might be a good idea if you found a day care for Stella. I hear good things about the facility at the Village Residence. What do you think?"

That was how I learned that Stella was beyond stage I.

5

The Right to Know

I picked up the address/telephone index and the whole A to Z gut cascaded — No! — out, a hundred sheets of names, phone numbers, addresses, some going back to before white-out, children tracked from dorm to apartment to house, friends from before tracked to vacation homes — Stop! Reverse gravity! — to nursing homes in Arizona and California, crossed out, deceased, written with pencils that happened to be there instead of the pen reached for; brain lobe of memory, uninsurable treasure picked up on the run out of the house on fire, that went on vacations with us — *No!*

Dealt from the edge of the table, collapsed to the floor, loose from the twelve-prong grab, pages with interleaved debris of business cards, return addresses torn from envelopes, recipes, saved postage stamps priced C and D — stupefying. But recoverable, not gone in the computer.

Bending to the rescue, as if speed made any difference now that it had happened — Take a breath. Light a cigar. Pour a drink — muttering curses on the universe — How could this happen? — I realized that Stella, sitting as close to the shocking event as I was, seemed not to be involved, seemed not surprised. After a glance at the flurry around me she had turned a page of her magazine. It implied complicity, foreknowledge.

"What happened here?"

"You dropped the address book."

"No, the inside fell out. Why was everything loose inside?"

"I don't know."

"Did you have pages out for any reason?"

"I think a few pages were out."

I think — speculating without exact knowledge. Pages were out — a natural phenomenon from which she was distanced. The disorder could not all have happened on the way to the floor. Alphabets were mixed. Pages had been torn from the metal fingers. Pages buried inside clumps were upside-down, frontside-back. I couldn't reconstruct the scene, but guessed enough. She had seen a name on a page, associated it with another name elsewhere, had torn out the page to bring them together, didn't get it right. Tore out more pages to remedy homeopathically what was not going well. I don't think Stella ever knew about opening the teeth of the spine by pressing an end. She wouldn't have thought about any technology after three-ring school binders. She was an artist, a musician, a lover, a mother who had been compelled by circumstances to master starting an automobile, aiming it, reading the gas gauge, going somewhere, and getting home. The blender and its clever tinware, used once, sat under a plastic tent in a corner of the kitchen counter.

Her patience and dexterity would have been challenged just to spread the prongs enough to slide in an extra S page without the whole section and a few Rs escaping like beagles through a cracked door. But there was nobody else, she must have done it. The sinewed hands of a cellist yanked at the teeth until they opened and everything came loose.

Her problem had ceased to be moving a page from here to there, had become a mess to put in order. She had gathered and arranged, squared edges fairly well, put it all back between covers (of course, not twelve metal fingers through the holes on a hundred sheets, some upside down, some backside front, Ks among Fs, Gs among Ms). Closed the book. The binder snapped at rows of punched holes, missed them all, and her instinct fell back to the ignorance of a child whose hand had been in the cookie jar. Or she may have forgotten whose hand. It may have happened as long ago as yesterday. Most likely, if remembered, it was without personal involvement, a scene in an old movie, a part in a play; not really herself.

"It's going to take me forever to get this together. Please don't take out any pages again."

"I didn't," she said.

I was getting used to Stella denying having anything to do with the mild disasters that trailed her: ringing telephones lifted from the hook and put down unanswered, spills, cap removed from toothpaste — where could a toothpaste cap be hidden in the bathroom? — and probably flushed away.

My status as caregiver was still a novelty. Only a few months before I had been only a husband, free to speak my mind as she was free to speak hers, within the rules for marriage we had discovered as we went along. I was still letting her know — anger well contained, but still letting her know — that although I was not holding her accountable, she had been caught creating chaos of the address book. I scored my points quietly, but I scored them, tongue bitten.

In his private time with Stella, Dr. Harrison had picked up this negative nuance when he probed for marital discord. The patient had said, "My husband is getting very upset with me . . . I'm slower in doing chores and have difficulty in remembering." It had shaken me to read "very upset." I had seen myself as scrupulously patient. "A little upset" was the most I would concede. However, we are not only what we think we are, we are what we are seen — or expected — to be. If Stella thought I had become adversarial, it was not enough to approach her slowly, palms uplifted, my intentions unmistakable. Stella had to see it as my natural bearing.

It took awhile. I had to get from what I knew in my head to what my nerves had to learn: there was no way to restore for any longer than the present moment the fraying connections in her brain. We could have a social conversation for a few moments about why a glass fell from her hand, but there could be no expectation that what I said, what she agreed to vaguely, would be born in mind. My first thought had to be that while the glass was still falling from her hand, before she could comprehend a lap full of orange juice and begin to account for it —

"Don't worry about it. It's just a spill. My fault, I shouldn't have left the glass there."

The point is not that I had developed a device for explaining such things away smoothly to contradict my churning stomach but that my emotions also now accepted the simple intellectual truth: the spill was in no way her fault. My stomach had learned to be no more concerned that she spilled juice than it was when an airplane took off and I continued to read or nap, oblivious of it.

To have a napkin to clean up, to tell her everything was okay, my fault, gave me far more relief than any fit of "When you pick up something, hold it!" punctuated with the slam punctuation as I might have a year before, without the slam a few months ago; and now, for as long as we go on, not saying or even thinking it. She had forgotten sequence, how to keep herself out of harm's way. It was up to me.

The next Christmas, packages showed up in our mail with dozens of cards she had ordered from Unicef, the Unitarian Service Committee, the Alzheimer's Association, museums of art — literally hundreds of cards. Her orders had escaped into the mail when I wasn't looking, probably dropped in the box by a helpful aide. I paid the bills and wrote them off as good causes. It was a miracle that she had written a few numbers, signed her name and stuck on our credit card label, gotten the pages in envelopes for a helpful aide to put in the box for the mailman to pick up. I sat with her and showed her cards. She always enjoyed cards, choosing them and receiving them.

BECAUSE the caregivers' group at the Alzheimer's Center was an adjunct to the patient group, when Stella drifted below stage 1 and had to be withdrawn, I also became homeless. It was during the frustrating months when she was between medications, waiting for her liver readings to return to normal.

While I maneuvered to get her on a productive medication at the clinic, I looked for new support groups. I couldn't imagine how a coed group that mingled caregivens and caregivers could be useful for both of us. Stella needed something to engage her mentally and socially and exercise her physically. I wanted time with other caregivers. I had trouble visualizing sitting beside Stella while a speaker went on about Alzheimer's . . . Alzheimer's . . . Alzheimer's, the kind of talk that could only arouse a useless anxiety in her. How would it profit her to sit through graphic descriptions of mental and physical disasters that were prospective for her and about which she could do nothing?

A day program sponsored by the senior center ten minutes from our front door was very much like the day care of childish drawings on the wall, of bingo and funny hats she had dismissed at a glance only months before. However, when we went to look CenterDay over I found that Stella had now, in a manner of speaking, grown into that kind of facility. She liked it. She liked the staff that welcomed her. I signed her in.

Although in some stage of depreciation and dependency, so that they no longer shopped unescorted or drove cars, the clients at CenterDay did not all have Alzheimer's. Typically, they lived with relatives who had major responsibility for them: children with jobs; sisters in good enough shape, one needing odds and ends of attention to get her through the days, both needing this brief respite from each other. The group went on excursions in the house bus to gardens and galleries. High-school choruses visited. The town banjo band played. Troubadors with penny whistles and harmonicas volunteered. "Who's for some artwork today?" a staff member asked with enthusiasm that drew affirmative answers. A client who had been a well-known local portrait artist soberly crayoned the blanks outlined in picture books. Another splashed colorful flowers on newspaper-size pages.

When they found out what music Stella liked to listen to, she was seated by the tape player in the corner for private concerts. Sometimes she fell asleep. I brought in a tape of a concert she had given and was impressed by the respect it received. That's Stell playing! It was a hard reminder that, without any evident traumatic event, she had lost the creative part of her life so quickly, recently, completely, irretrievably. The last time I had brought her cello to her and urged her hand to take the bow, she had grasped it, smiled amiably, and let it rub slackly down the strings to the floor.

The program spelled out in the center's brochure was of little importance compared to the vitality of the staff. Stella was not the only bingo player they found the numbers for and told when to hold up a winner's hand. In this sense, all of CenterDay was bingo writ large: The importance of the experience was not the activities but being in the midst of something going on, if only as observer. When asked at home if it had been a good day for her, Stella invariably said it had, which the staff confirmed and I observed when I dropped in.

Mornings began with an extra breakfast of Danish and juice, then sedentary exercises in circled chairs — a beach ball kicked back and forth in the ring, a lot of Simon Says. A man with a willing baritone led Irish songs. Headlines in the morning paper were reviewed, animal pictures scissored from magazines were pasted in albums. In all this, Stella participated only as an observer. Time out for toileting. Lunch was the robust meal published in the monthly calendar. I respect nutritionists who plan meals thirty days ahead, down to the kind of gravy. For me, the deli departments of the markets are satisfactory resources for salads, sandwich fillings, chickens from slices to the whole broiled beast. My chef's specials — baked apples, elementary pasta, and a couple of soups — tend to become boring with repetition.

Even when Stella had been a proficient cook, she had asked me for suggestions about dinner. I had wondered how choosing dinner could be a problem with all those cookbooks. The cookbook shelf was as wide as the kitchen wall. I inherited the paradox of a house with a card file of recipes, forty cookbooks and not one good idea for dinner tonight.

As Stella, on day-program days, had her main meal at noon at the center, I had mine from the refrigerator or at a downtown saloon. Serious dining at noon, like dinner at four, was a farmer's schedule. For evening meals we went more frequently to friends and restaurants. Grita kept us a casserole ahead and dressed up meals on her duty days with gravies, roasted potatoes, salads with the right herbs.

When the children visited, the kitchen became a bazaar of ethnic and generational cooking, strangely spiced Far and Middle Eastern vegetables, pastes, and gravies; European puddings and breads; Jewish soups; Italian pastas; Malaysian, African, and Scandinavian stews. In spite of holding responsible jobs with time out only to begin their families, Marion and Connie were throwbacks beyond their mothers, to their grandmothers. They tasted in their heads, kept an oven and three pots timed to the minute.

Unlike me, Damon and Jerry were of a generation of husbands who disdained store-bought pesto and made ten-ingredient lentil soups. Despite stir-fries on the burner and ringing phones, they heard the day's adventures of children more attentively than we — at least I — had heard theirs.

WHILE Stella had three half-days a week at CenterDay and on other days was at home with Grita or another aide, I was free to work at my desk or in the garden, see a movie, take an hour at the library, or lunch with friends, and I looked for caregiver groups to sit in with, especially small groups of my caregiving peers, much like the one I had been obliged to leave when Stella passed from stage 1, in which practical knowledge was shared. Meetings in which authorities stood at a podium and talked at me and answered questions sent up from the floor were not my idea of support groups; but authorities did know about research and legislation and occasionally I went to hear them. I was in the audience for a visiting genius whose subject was "The Right to Know." I wrote down one passage as he said it:

> Any handicapped person is due a full explanation of his or her condition. They have a right to know. His or her caregiver or doctor should take the time to provide a full explanation so they can participate in the decision-making process.

I was unlikely to take much guidance from anybody who did not know how to extricate himself from a morass of hises, hers, and theys. It implied that he was repeating jargon and clichés without having thought the process through to its meaning in anybody's real life.

Stella's right to know was not an abstraction to me. The first time she asked me if I thought she might have Alzheimer's I felt challenged to the root of the trusting relationship we had had for so many years. Not lying to each other was the unspoken compact between individuals of equal powers, equal responsibilities. But had the weight not shifted? Was I not supposed to compensate in some way? I chose to hear not Alzheimer's but *might*.

"Yes, sure. I may have it too. Many cases are genetic. It hides in the cells and emerges bit by bit, if at all, in elderly people. The older we are — at our age, yours and mine — the less likely it is ever to appear in its severest form. It isn't ever possible to say absolutely that anybody has Alzheimer's. It's only an educated guess. All anybody knows are symptoms. It isn't a disease with germs they can see under a microscope."

Every word was true, but she couldn't relate to any of it, and only my "Yes, sure" was forthcoming. She would not have taken the question to another level: Exactly what is it? A wasting, incurable disease. It isn't painful. You may not even be aware of it except as a vague inconvenience. How will it affect me? It will destroy your ability to think, to speak, to control functions, and perhaps to walk. What do I do about it? Nothing from the inside. I am outside it and will do whatever helps you live at peace with it. What are the odds? For recovery, none. For living with it comfortably, we'll have to see. You may just lose a little more memory from time to time. You can live with that. It may be more severe. You may become incontinent, wheelchair-bound, forget how to chew or swallow, want to sleep all the time, be unable to speak. You may take it in stride, step-by-step. Or you may become profoundly unhappy, depressed, suicidal, and need drugs to even want to get up in the morning. Whatever it is, you can't do a thing about it. What habits do I change? Your habits will decide for themselves which persist, which are lost. What provisions should I make in my will? You and I have done all that. Our lists of things we would like done, people we want something special for are with our wills. The children know all about it. If you want to read your will again someday, I'll get it out of the file for you. If there is anything you want to change, tell me.

What earthly good could have come of more than a few of those words, except to satisfy some theory-ridden pamphleteer that his misguided notion of human rights had fallen into the hands of somebody foolish enough to confront his wife with her right to know, and, if he was sufficiently graphic, needlessly scare her half to death?

Many people with Alzheimer's retain the ability and have the temperament and will to control their remaining options — to drive, to write checks, to shop, to take a walk, to feed birds — although this control may diminish with little or no warning. They retain capacities. Rights are useful to them. Rights are their due, an affirmation of their humanity and their continued participation in society.

Stella, on the other hand, had passed almost instantly to a condition in which she was unable to discriminate between her right to be informed and their right to require her signature. The very statement of difference had no meaning for her.

In what consultation about blood tests and chest X rays or billing was her input essential? What meaningful instruction about Alzheimer's was it her right to receive, the doctor's to impart, and her signature to confirm? What part of the decision-making process was she to participate in on any basis except the smarmy, "Let's see now, what shall we do about this? Shall we sign our name here?" The intelligent well knew that the essence of the "rights transaction" was the patient's signature on forms that in a crunch were intended to make it appear that she had competently signed them away.

From the beginning, the last thing I wanted was for Dr. Loughrand to blunder through an interview with Stella explaining what Alzheimer's might do to her. Insistent fore-knowledge would not prepare her for anything in which the primary components would be helplessness and forgetting. Loughrand owed me, not her, his knowledge. I thought the same of Geerey the neurologist and Harrison the psychiatrist.

The durable power of attorney I held was exercisable at my discretion. It was not symbolic. Her right to depend on me transcended rights prescribed by somebody commissioned to produce a pamphlet. "Loughrand told you, it can look like stroke for a while. It often can look like depression, and you certainly aren't depressed. Do you feel depressed? Really down in the dumps? If you do, I don't see it." I did not say "suicidal." This was not an exercise in candor but in feeling.

"Do I feel that way? Of course not."

Stella had heard as much lecture-talk as she cared for and withdrew her attention. When she asked again at another time, I reprised and added that the only way they knew anybody had Alzheimer's was by drilling deep into the brain and looking at the condition of the nerves. That isn't something you do on living subjects. It's done at autopsy. Was she so anxious to find out that she wanted them drilling into her brain?

"Good God no."

As time passed she had even less curiosity and cared even less to endure technical explanations. What she needed to know, when she asked why we were going to this clinic or that doctor or why she took these pills and another blood test, was not that we were treating Alzheimer's but that we were trying different medicines to see which might help her walk steadier, remember better, and not give her hepatitis as a side effect. Those were the tangible, comprehensible details. Those were the questions I spoke to.

I was adept at changing the channel when I thought the program might get into Alzheimer's. I pulled out suspect pages before handing her newspapers. I did not think she absorbed information effectively, but I did not want to risk a moment when there might dawn on her an image of herself helpless and incontinent, belted to a chair in a nursing home.

Other caregivers see the issue of candor differently and agree with the speaker who advocated the right to know. Awkward grammar is by itself not a good reason to reject what may be good advice. From what I heard in support groups, others with Alzheimer's are aggressive in finding out what is the matter with them and cannot be turned aside as readily as Stella. Were one of them my ward, I would go along as far as she took me, giving as much answer as she could use; which was what I did for Stella. The reality was that she could use very little.

SHAM creeps into the well-intended. What did it prove about autonomy to have Stella's signature on documents when her hand had been guided by mine?

What does even my signature prove when a hospital presents a sheaf of documents to be signed forthwith or I will be denied the services of a surgeon, an anesthetist, in fact the whole institution? If you don't like it, what can you do about it? Refuse anesthesia? Refuse to have your blood tested? The next hospital presents the same boilerplate papers. Nobody reads. Everybody signs. The papers are presented for instant signature in an environment of "Everybody does it, it's only a form." The patient's right to sign or not has the color of blackmail. Responsibility, except the patient's, is never in the room. The compelling party waves back toward the lawyers or the insurance company as the initiator.

In most hospitals and larger nursing homes and health management organizations an employee is designated to be something called patient representative or patient advocate or even ombudsperson. The question sometimes arises: do they represent patients to management or management to patients? Whose interest is primary? A simple test is to ask one of them to get the papers revised to describe what rights the patient is not being asked to sign away.

It is a great mystery that hard-won rights embedded in law — free speech, trial rights, defenses against faulty products and services — can be signed away at all, by anybody, competent or not. Have we the right to work for less than the minimum wage? Can we sign ourselves into servitude if a keen administrator sees it as a way to make his life easier? I understand that the patient's signature is part of the package that comes with the empowering of the disadvantaged, but to require assent from people who cannot meaningfully give it is contrary to the purpose of right and trivializes it.

Once when my back was turned, a medical technician procured Stella's scrawled initials needed to set up an improper billing for a service that should not have been rendered. It took a lot of going through channels to get the apologetic letter and the fake transaction off my credit report. They kept telling me they had her signature on the order, and I kept telling each higher level of review, "Pay attention! The signer has Alzheimer's. It was known to the clerk who solicited her signature. It is not even a signature, it is an initial and the scrawl of an undirected pen."

Eventually I arrived before a sane judge and had $160 to show for more letters and hours of advocacy than I should admit to, considering that I hadn't the time for any of it. Nevertheless, I do not regret it, and I urge you to spend your energy disproportionately to defend against such aggravating abuses as come your way. Not enough of us go the course.

In the long run, the caregiver is custodian of the patient's rights. What Stella personally retained, while it is not affirmative, is a kind of veto in her area of competence: what she likes or dislikes, what she feels. In this, her house, it is her "right." She cannot say what she would like for dinner, but if food displeases her, she will turn away from it. In this way she tells caregivers not to offer string beans; but if they are the green vegetable of the day, it is all right to puree them and embed them in applesauce. We don't say what was, to our advantage, said to us by our parents when we were learning beings: "Eat what is in front of you or go to bed hungry."

She is almost completely without complaint of physical discomfort, but if asked whether she is warm enough, her answer is a firm and reliable yes or no. Actual pain — if her skin is inadvertently pinched when she is being transferred from bed to chair — is revealed in an unostentatious yelp. Without having any intent to test it, I believe that if I told her she had to endure a painful medical procedure without an anesthetic she would suffer it well if I stayed with her and kept reassuring. As for her other rights, it is up to her caregivers and aides to perceive her needs and fulfill them as best they can.

The visiting genius had it all wrong for Stella, but for me, he was essentially correct: If I come to Alzheimer's, I want the candor I reject for my wife. I have the right to know because I have thought about it and said ahead of the decision that I want to know. When the lab nurse aimed the needle at her vein, Stella always turned away. I watch. I count the vials of blood drawn. I want to know why three; two were enough last time. Stella never knew whether they drew one or five.

I also know, having seen Alz up close, that there may come a time in the course of the disease when the concept of candor may fade from my intellect as the boundaries of the real and the imaginary fade. Candor may become for me as irrelevant as it has for Stella. I will not know it when I hear it.

If I come to the condition where my caregivers judge that I no longer understand true from kindly intended false, in the same implied oath with which I now require their candor I absolve them from it. I will no longer have the right to know. They have my permission, given when my mind is as sound as it is ever going to be, to lie to me then. If it is the judgment of my son and daughter that processes have little meaning for me, it is their call to make. A time came when the word Alzheimer's gradually became a not especially noticed part of Stella's culture. It ceased to have a special sound. Benign censorship was no longer needed. I couldn't say exactly when the disease began, and I couldn't say when the word ceased to carry the little freight it had had for her since she first failed the Sevens.

Not only conversations about Alzheimer's but all talk going on around her unrelated to an act in which she was involved ceased to hold her attention. She dozed not only through Alzheimer's but through Red Sox, Guerilla Warfare in Mexico, Garden Club Elects New Officers, War on Drugs, Mozart. We no longer blacked out subjects, and not because she was rudely assumed not to be in the conversation. She remained very much present to me, but I knew that some subjects no longer engaged her; they had no history, no vital present, neither reward nor menace.

Certainly it is a transgression to speak around a person, to act as if she is a child who hasn't enough vocabulary or educated instinct to understand. In an Alzheimer patient it is especially unjustified to assume that what she cannot say she must not know. Stella gave many evidences that much that went on around her had meaning for her long after she lost the vocabulary to deal with it. But there came a time when certain words and ideas lost their force so that they hardly seeped into her consciousness, a lightbulb giving too little light to read by. Words like *Alzheimer's* that proved themselves to be without meaning no longer had to be avoided. It was a somewhat backward restoration of the accustomed candor to our marriage.

An exception I never understood was how attentive she remained to intelligent discourse on television. Customarily, I surf the channels, pausing at candidates for her attention and asking, "This one? Do you want to watch this movie? This ballgame? These insects mating? This talk show?" I often run our sixty-eight channels and find nothing to interest her. Her negatives range from a bored tilt of her head, to merely closing her eyes, to a murmured no, to emphatic *no!* when we come to gunplay movies or shows that feature apparently intelligent panelists shouting at each other. She has better sense than they have; she prefers to sit quietly or doze. She accepts mute golf, perhaps for the scenery, or a ballgame if nothing else is on.

It is when I get to something like a book review that she is most likely to say "yes" and often stays with it for a considerable distance. One evening early in her fourth Alzheimer's year, Stella did not take her eyes from the screen during successive half-hour biographies of Melville, Thoreau, and Whitman. I marveled at her concentration.

She could not tell me one word of what she had been watching. Can I say therefore that she did not have a real relationship to what happened on the screen?

6

The Real and the Unreal

Of the more than two thousand caregiver groups around the country with support and sponsorship from regional chapters of the Alzheimer's Association, a dozen were in my county. They met in senior centers, in churches and temples, in town halls, in nursing homes and private homes, in basements of banks.

One had a fixed agenda, an announced subject for each meeting, visiting speakers, readers, and a fixed entry date, like a college course, so that all members who attended regularly had about the same level of information.

Most groups were structured less formally and met only once or twice a month, the membership being those who happened to be present, with a core of three or four who came regularly to meet friends who had caregiving in common. I first settled into one that had no formal structure except its meeting date in the library of a nursing home on the third Thursday of every month. I joined by showing up and saying a few words to introduce myself when the facilitator said, "Let's get started."

"My name is Aaron Alterra. My wife is in her second year of Alzheimer's. Maybe third. I don't know how much of the beginning I missed. She is cared for at home. We have some home aide time. Three days a week she goes to the center for their day program, which she enjoys very much."

When groups met, as we did, at a nursing home, most of the caregivers had relatives who lived there and the facilitator was a staff person. Some members had been dropping in for years. They knew each other's histories. They did not come to learn anything about Alzheimer's. They knew quite enough. Repetition did not seem to bother them. They came for the understanding companionships that had developed over time. They knew the names of each other's spouses and asked about them. Obituaries were of people they knew. The agenda of such groups was mostly to provide fellowship.

Freed of the requirement that caregiven and caregiver be paired, the natural gender distribution of caregivers became evident. There were seldom more than one or two men in the average group of a half dozen. Dan Boudreau, the pharmaceutical route salesman who had been with me in Ina's group migrated here after Alma had been signed out by Lenore, dispossessing him from Ina's cadre of spouses. He came regularly. It was his club.

The disadvantage of the open door for somebody like me who was not especially looking for companionship or occupation, as I had more than enough of both for my interests, was that the meetings kept going over well-traveled ground. Newcomers came in with classic questions: How do you get them to stop driving? What medication is he on? What if she wanders away when nobody is looking?

I moved from group to group. Most groups met only an hour or two every month. In several groups it was possible to show up once or twice a year and thereafter be thought of as a regular who happened to miss a meeting or two. Each of us was at one time a newcomer, introducing himself and the relationship he had to a person with Alzheimer's, mentioning something about wandering, or hallucinating, or driving, offered as a casual interjection in an otherwise normal life, or as a horrendous new experience. "I am going out of my mind. She is off like a shot with no warning. . ."

The facilitator says, "Of all immediate reasons people with Alzheimer's come to nursing homes, the family's inability to cope with intractable wandering may be the most frequent."

We know AJ's story and that he will tell it. His sister wandered away several times before he had the house wired to warn if it happened again. Black carpet at exits implied bottomless pits, best to avoid. Still, she once slipped the defenses and walked miles from home to the next town and the town after that, on country roads and highways, sleeping no one knew where, leaving a caring home (who always knows what the ill think is caring?) for no apparent goal, lost to the police until she sat in bewilderment in the aisle of a shopping mall. More likely the wanderer is in a strange neighborhood a mile from home, unnoticed until somebody hesitantly calls 911.

Someone has a clipping of a new satellite search service that can track members to within thirty feet anywhere in the world. Somebody says, "That's for J. Paul Getty." Somebody says, "They put out those stories to entertain reporters. In a million years they'll get around to the real world."

Stella never wandered from home, but if I left her at the entrance of the supermarket and said, "Please stay right there while I park the car, I'll be back in a minute," I might see her in the rearview ambling in the direction I had driven. In the market, momentarily out of my sight, she might lag into an aisle. Amble and lag were her pace, she never set off with the drive that takes many wanderers out of their neighborhoods.

The woman who was going out of her mind says, "I never before thought of being confined to a wheelchair as a blessing."

The facilitator gives her the association's Safe Return pamphlet. The association has identification bracelets and necklaces and ties with local police and a national network. From the collective experience of the group, different kinds of locking devices and barriers are suggested.

We have the peculiar intimacy of isolated strangers, like passengers on overnight flights who fall into conversation. After a short time we won't see each other again. The circumstance of being in the same situation may lead some of us to tell an excess of truth in order to engage each other, but I don't think any of my friends here err on the side of reticence. If a subject comes up, there is an obligation to disclose. As the nurses in our Alzheimer's patients' lives realize more than doctors, we caregivers know more than nurses and academics. We live it.

We tell our favorite stories to comfort those who haven't been there yet, or maybe we become raconteurs only to define ourselves as individuals for them. Somebody remembers leaving her aunt seat-belted in a locked car for "no time at all" and returned to find her (or not find her) gone, like Houdini. Somebody else remembers the day her husband lost the car keys, got the spare keys from the rack in the kitchen and lost them too; both sets were found in the breast pocket of the suit he was wearing. Somebody else comments with one of the standard Alzheimer's tenets: "They aren't in real trouble until they forget what keys are for."

I am likely to tell the story of the day Stella and I were driving through Pennsylvania on the way to visit her sister. It was soon after her Alzheimer's had been diagnosed. Stella had stopped driving and I had turned in her license. I pulled off four-lane Interstate 80 at a dot on the map to call ahead to the motel to let them know our arrival time.

"I'm only going to make a phone call to the motel. I'll be back in a couple of minutes. Stay in the car. I'll be right back."

I was beginning to give such instructions firmly and repetitively. I didn't expect her to wander away — she never wandered as I understood wandering: Doing something purposeful in order to be somewhere else. However, she drifted. In an art museum with several floors and many galleries she had vanished from my side. Guards found her at the end of a maze of corridors and rooms. The galleries were not confusingly busy. Inasmuch as I was the responsible party, it would be more exact to say I had lost her rather than the other way around. She certainly hadn't run away. She hadn't planned.

And when she ambled on my trail after I dropped her off at a supermarket or movie and asked her to wait while I parked, I hadn't thought of it as wandering; wandering was *away* in my mind, Stella was going *toward*. Alzheimer's lurched through her in fits and starts in those early months, and I was never ahead of it, but always chasing after, trying to be where it was taking her. Eventually I applied for a handicapped parking placard that assured us a place near the door.

When I completed the brief call to the motel and returned to the street she was gone. The car was gone. She wouldn't know where she was. She would have no idea where she was going. She wouldn't be able to explain driving without a license. I had read about car hijackers who showed women a knife, told them to move over and drove away with them. She had also forgotten how to raise her voice for any reason. At home, she couldn't call me from an adjoining room. I had coached her on how to call for help, a voice therapist had also tried, but "Help me!" came out as mildly as asking for salt.

I wheeled back into the store and called the police. The cruiser was there in a few seconds. I told the officer what was going on.

He was puzzled. "She just drove away?"

Yes, I assumed so. I didn't mention carjackers. This little town wasn't the place for such a bizarre event. Hijacking was a big city or a big mall parking lot stunt.

"I wasn't gone more than two minutes."

"Why would she drive away?"

I didn't know. She hadn't been well.

"Did you have an argument?"

No, no. Nothing like that. Couldn't we talk later? Now we needed an all-points call, including the state police, to look for a car driven by a woman who had no license, who was ill, who could not really drive, who was in great danger and endangered others. She might be pulling off the ramp onto Interstate 80, bewildered, going at half the expected speed, surrounded, and overrun by roaring tractor trailers headed for the horizon.

"It isn't usual for a woman to drive away and leave her husband unless she wants to get away from him. You didn't have words with her?"

If he hadn't had a gun I might have been more vehement, and then, like a true cop, men of tender feeling, he would have forgotten everything but my disrespect. I would have confirmed his suspicion that I, not my wife, needed his attention. He would have booked me and addressed the wife problem later. The gun told me he was in charge and in an even voice I pressed the need to put out a call. Reluctantly he radioed the details: the license, the state, make of car, color, year, description of the woman, why the car should be stopped, who should be notified. He kept the radio crackling and said, "Let's drive around and look."

I got in beside him and we drove the only main street. He soon pointed into a parking strip in front of a row of stores.

"Is that your car? Is that your wife?"

My car! My wife! I thanked him and ran to her. He was right beside me, doing his duty.

"Where have you been?" Stella asked, the image of the injured wife. "I've been waiting and waiting."

I don't think that the cop quite believed I had parked where I said I had, that I hadn't had an argument with her. I might slap her as soon as he turned his back. At the station house he would tell the others that he should have brought me in, held me until it was straightened out, called my hometown police to see if I had a record, booked me to teach me a lesson.

The officer's skepticism was not radically different from Dr. Harrison's. I concede they both came at me with the right professional attitude. Testimony in favor of ourselves always sounds a little contrived. Harrison was right to be skeptical without more evidence that a disease and not her husband was his new patient's main problem. The cop was right to suspect that her husband had done away with her; that he was trying to create a cover story; that she would be in the trunk of the car when it was found.

As the same questions come up and the same stories are told and the police are called and the disappearances are like Houdini's, the main reason to be in the group becomes companionship. I confess that while I fully understand the need for that kind of support, I am content to have the few friends I have and spend my recreation time reading a book or transplanting bushes. For that reason, I seldom gave more than a few weeks to any group before moving on to one that may have something newer to say to me and I to them. I recycle back when I think there has been time for some old stories to have retired.

A GROUP met in the basement of a bank. There were six of us. It was my first day and I arrived early, having misunderstood the convening time by fifteen minutes. The other group members and the facilitator straggled in. They all knew each other from before and warmly commiserated with a woman whose husband had died that week. It was in the paper.

I became aware that a woman nobody knew had taken a seat and had not been as forward as I had been in socializing. It was almost as if she had materialized behind the screen of the others. I live in a resort area and by their particular kind of stylishness some women are immediately identifiable as summer people. She was around fifty, a little old for the narrow velvet ribbon that bound her hair. Her sandals were of finely woven leather. She was almost certainly summering in a cottage at the golf and tennis inn or in a house on the peninsula. From here she would go back to a good address in New York City or Rochester and, after Thanksgiving or the Christmas holidays, to Palm Beach or Naples and more golf, scotch whisky, a boat with a canopy. More than half her life ago, she would have finished her academic years in Lausanne or at a woman's college in the Yale dating orbit. None of this may have been true, but it was the story told by her demeanor and the clothes she wore.

"And you are — ?" the facilitator asked her gently.

She didn't want to give up her name but did. It was Daisy. She was out of F. Scott Fitzgerald.

The facilitator waited an instant for more that was not forthcoming.

"You are a caregiver for — your mother? An aunt? Your husband?" Daisy was young to have a contemporary husband with Alzheimer's but she hadn't taken up her options on the other choices.

"I read about this group in the newspaper. I thought you might be able to tell me if, that is, if my husband has some Alzheimer's."

Nobody had ever heard such a question. People who had a family member with Alzheimer's knew it already. They didn't come to groups for diagnoses. Gears shifted inside the imperturbable facilitator. "We may not have the answers you are looking for, but let's see. Does somebody say he has Alzheimer's?"

"The doctor seems to think so. I didn't talk to him. He told my husband he might have a touch of Alzheimer's."

A touch. Something to get over, like the flu. "Was something bothering your husband that caused him to talk to a doctor?"

"I said I thought he should see a doctor. He was forgetting things like appointments. And he thought there were people living upstairs. Of course there weren't."

"Of course."

Somebody upstairs, the most common hallucination. Not unexpected, not disquieting — somebody upstairs. From caregivers I have heard horrendous hallucinations of blistering fires, spouses hallucinating falls from buildings in screaming panic, dead parents who return with instructions that cause daughters to search frantically in desk drawers, communists coming down from the attic. Most hallucinations I hear of, however, are benign.

Hours — sometimes days — after overnight guests said good-bye, Stella matter-of-factly said they are upstairs, maybe they would come down for dinner. We have no upstairs in our house; she meant downstairs. Their images lingered. "The Shavitzes never come out of their room. I never see them." For Stella, events of scattered time became photos in an accordion file that folded to the image of the one on top.

I rebelled at the received wisdom that it was best to be agreeable when your loved one hallucinated. I didn't make a point of correcting her but I did say that it wasn't likely, I thought they had gone home. I don't know if by this I was declining to demean her or myself by condoning nonsense. Probably it was self-serving; Stella was not concerned with whether they were with us or had gone. She had no expectations to fulfill, no plans for them. Her life had become more pageant than engagement, except when it was immediate and vivid, like a glass of water.

Much that is called hallucination is simply lack of vocabulary. If *up* becomes *down* and *there* becomes *here,* it is understandable that *absent* becomes *present.* Stella seemed to mean *that* she has experienced a happening, not *where* or *when*. An analogy would be a primitive civilization that had only one word for every kind of cover from weather — tent, cave, hole in the ground, hat, umbrella, all the same. It would take a while for a visitor to understand what to make of a man who lived in his hat.

When she still had whole sentences, she had asked her sister, "How is Dad?" when he had been dead for twenty years. "I got a letter from him yesterday." Going through an album of old photographs and letters she may have seen something that remained with her as presence.

Last year, in one of those phases that have their short moment — like getting into the car once with the wrong foot forward — television announcers addressed her personally. She knew them from having seen them before, they deserved answers. There were brief dialogues between Stella and Sam Donaldson. They no longer occur.

Sometimes what seemed to be irrational (which would require Yes to the clinic's monthly question, Does the patient experience hallucinations?) was a simple mistake of observation reported by an inadequate vocabulary. When she said she had seen Jack Nicklaus playing golf on our lawn, she had seen the TV image of the golfer reflected in the window that overlooks our side yard. Such illusions are actual in the sense that movies are actual — actually on the screen and at the same time they lack ultimate conviction. Those were the kinds of hallucinations Stella had. She had no commitment to them. They were movies, pageants, mostly of real events that had been compressed in time, gender, direction, and language to a hallucinate dimension.

When at check-up time at the clinic they opened the ring binders to the hallucination page and asked if Stella had any, I dutifully reported and they recorded. I did not impose my theories on them. They had enough of their own. They made their notes and turned the page to another subject.

From senior physician to receptionist, from medical technician to case chief, the clinic staff is consistently courteous and attentive, but I bear in mind that they are there to accumulate a research record for a multibillion-dollar firm that wants to convince the FDA that it has a safe and useful drug to market. The clinic is not there to encourage or discourage hallucinations; it is there to dispense medicine, to record, to fill in data on a curve.

Hallucinating was a passing phase. It may be that Stella's ordinary consciousness is so replete with transferences that we do not even recognize when she is engrossed by one. How would we know? As she no longer has what would be called dialogue with her family, although there is extensive communication, she may be interacting with Oprah as she does with us. Scenery on TV may be as real to her as her own outdoors. If no capacities are restored in Alzheimer's, how does discrimination between the real and the hallucinatory become a significant exception?

THE facilitator of our caregivers group uses whatever is offered. So Daisy's husband hallucinated?

"Does your husband drive?" Nobody is indulged for hallucinating in traffic.

"Oh yes."

"Does he drive well? Has there been a change in the way he drives?"

"Not much. He likes to have me with him when he goes anywhere. He likes me to drive. People are quite different and it takes some time to get used to each other. We have been married only two years."

"Of course," the facilitator said to keep her going.

"The doctor said he thought he had fourth stage Alzheimer's."

One of the old hands could not contain herself, "Nobody who is fourth stage is driving an automobile!" Stage IV is helpless in a wheelchair, not knowing your children! The doctor should be brought up on charges to the medical society.

The facilitator heard garble. "Perhaps he said first stage? We don't always hear unfamiliar things exactly."

Daisy agreed that was possible. She matched the facilitator's imperturbability but she had shown her hand. She knew nothing. I had never before seen a caregiver who seemed not to have the least idea of what was going on. Two years married and her husband thought somebody was upstairs and she had just begun to wonder.

The facilitator brought out two narrow brochures. "Take these. There may be something in there for you. We'll talk later." She turned her attention to the woman whose husband had died.

One hour passes quickly. The facilitator looked at her watch. "I guess it's time. See you again the second Wednesday."

We got to our feet slowly, with sidebar conversations, and Daisy slipped out as quietly as she had come in. Not a word had been said to her since she had taken the pamphlets. The facilitator realized there was unfinished business and thought to hold on to her, but she would be talking to Daisy's back.

She had come with her question about Alzheimer's and the husband she did not know very well. Was she really that dumb? I had asked that of myself when for months Stella had Alzheimer's and I didn't recognize it. Had she heard enough to last her for a while? Had she noticed something in one of the pamphlets?

Moving with all deliberate speed, like a man who intends to get to the head of the line without being showy about it, I set out to intercept her on the stairs or in the parking lot. Her car was an old, still dapper, two door, the kind you leave behind on blocks at the end of summer and pick up again next year. I held up a finger to hold her attention.

"I don't want to butt in. The facilitator would have said something useful to you if you hadn't gotten away —"

She was wary. For a moment I had the ridiculous vanity that she would think I was making a move on her. What she was looking at, though, was somebody older than her father, unshaven, wearing an open collar denim shirt with an ink-stained breast pocket, wrinkled pants, moccasins; a local stray.

I asked if she knew the Alzheimer's Association office in Hyannis. She relaxed a little.

"I don't think I do."

"The address and phone will be on those pamphlets. Try to talk to Ina Krillman. She'll answer all your questions and give you all the time you want."

"Well thank you very much," she said, meaning, Thank you some.

"Do you mind my asking if you have some family to share this with?"

"Not really. I have no children and Hugh's didn't," she decided to trust my anonymity, more likely than my probity, "didn't exactly approve of his marrying again. They don't keep in touch much." She said it flatly, without regret, describing the situation as it was.

"That's too bad, but those things work out," if by working out I meant there is always something next, which can be said until world's end. "See Ina. She is experienced and understanding. You can talk to her."

I know she did that because I asked Ina. By then it was after Labor Day and Daisy's season would be over. Ina didn't let any confidences out but she added to what I already knew. "I suggested she see a doctor as soon as she got back to Rochester and push to get her husband on medication as soon as possible when there is a real diagnosis. I gave her our office number in Rochester."

I asked, "Do you think she'll cave in and walk away from the marriage?"

"I don't know. I wouldn't blame her, but my impression is she can be one tough cookie. Not likely to cave in, but she could make a deliberate decision, which is something else. I'm not the one to judge that. I do think that since we talked she knows what she may be in for."

I DID not return to that group for several months and had forgotten about Daisy until she came in, not anonymously as before but as a familiar who knew the others. Having been sure she was long gone, I was surprised to see her. Without indicating that we had met, she took the vacant chair next to mine. Conversations began, and I pieced together what the others knew. She had made hard choices, in a sense all the more difficult because Hugh retained enough competence to do many things for himself and resisted her efforts to deal with his losses. She had decided to live year-round on the Cape where there were people to talk to.

The conversation turned to wandering, one of the canon subjects. Wandering stories were told. Daisy said Hugh never wandered. He became disoriented, didn't know where he was, but he stayed home, never wandered. I waited to hear what the others probably knew — was he still driving? — but it did not come out.

"He will wander," one of the women said.

"He won't go out without me," Daisy said. "When I'm out he waits for me to come home. He won't go off the porch." She could have been speaking of a Labrador retriever.

"He will wander," the woman said again. Another asked, "Does he have a Safe Return bracelet?"

"No. He doesn't need it."

"They all wander," the woman said, and the other said, "He will wander."

Daisy was being badgered and the facilitator was letting it play out. I found myself saying, "Maybe yes, maybe no. Every case is different."

"That's so," the facilitator agreed, and turned us toward a new pamphlet she had from the association.

When the session ended, I stood, and backed my chair from the table to make room for Daisy. She got up in a flow of motion that I expected to be completed by her continuing to turn until she faced toward the door and went out. Instead, she stopped when we faced each other, hardly an arm's length apart, and examined my face, inch by inch it seemed, beginning with my eyes, seeing, as a magnifying mirror sees, where my beard began and ended, that my lips were thin and wide, that my ears were close to my head (maybe even knowing enough to guess double mastoid surgery when I was very young) and coming back unhurried to my eyes. Of necessity I did the same to her. It was not the face I would have remembered from the parking lot, the product of a particular kind of post-deb, country club life, the myth of my own invention jogged into existence by the velvet headband. Expressed in the face I now saw was what Ina had seen in Daisy and I had missed.

"Thank you," she said; whether for standing aside, suggesting Ina to her, or taking her part in the well-meant inquisition about wandering, I don't know, as not another word passed between us and I never saw her again. Psychologically, we expect something more from a narrative, but life as it is lived is full of brief encounters that leave lasting impressions.

Vincent Devlin also disappeared after a few meetings. His wife was in the Alz wing of the nursing home. Vin may have been on the edge of Alz himself. He had been headmaster of a school in Connecticut and, to his own frequent amusement, lived in a ruin of intellect and vocabulary. Words got away from him. He would pause and stretch his jaw down to where what he was looking for might be, regretting that he tried our patience while he searched. Plausible words that were not quite what he had in mind appeared in his mouth. I was empathetic to that as something that happened to me too. He reported that his wife's new disability was apnea in the knee.

"Apnea in the knee?" repeated the facilitator, reaching for ground. A knee that had a breathing problem —

"Yes — oh no, no, no," Vin laughed, opening his hands toward me in a wry petition to be excused. "Edema, I mean edema. Her knee is swollen."

I had an instinctive liking for him, and by the way he directed his comments and apologies I understood that he had singled me out as — in the imaginative concept of Kurt Vonnegut — a member of his karass. Not a club or church or neighborhood, nothing to put your finger on, just the sense of chance acquaintances — contrary to rationality — that we had known each other in a prior life. I visualized that his wife had as little self-awareness as Stella, while Vin was fully aware that he himself was going down, how fast or toward what he could not foresee, and that he would be far gone before he relinquished his insight.

I thought that from my experience I might be helpful to him as no priest or doctor could, but before I got around to it, one day he wasn't there. We convened only once a month, another absence was needed to confirm that he was no longer with us. The facilitator said she understood that the Devlins had decided to move to the Midwest to be near a caring daughter. I sent him a note to say he was missed and wishing him well. Whether he got it or not I don't know, I didn't hear from him. The nature of caregiver groups is that they go on with a freight of constantly changing innocents like Daisy and Vin and me, who become knowledgeable, often when what we come to know is no longer useful to ourselves, but may have a half-life remaining for others.

7

ANOTHER WAY

Dining-out evenings became dining-in as difficulties with spoons and forks and walking compounded. Crossing a restaurant floor, walking the flagstones to the door of a friend's house became too much. Without a clue in the blood work from the lab, without the traumatic turning point of a midnight run in the ambulance, she passed in a few months from needing only an occasional hand to halting Geisha steps, feeling for footing as if fording a stream on mossy rocks. Her feet never left the floor. I thought of Antaeus as a man of my age with Alzheimer's, otherwise in good shape.

Monday she knew how to brush her teeth. Tuesday she didn't. When the road is blocked, the healthy look for another way. Our habit is to think that if there is no recovery from injury, muscles and nerves learn a good enough detour to the same destination. We practice with the opposite hand. The person with Alzheimer's hasn't the resources to find a way around; that task is left to the caregiver.

As she looked at the brush and toothpaste tube as objects for which there was no known use, I put paste on the brush and placed the handle in her hand. "Time to brush your teeth, Stell." I might as well have handed her Rubik's cube. Urging her resistant hand upward I got the brush to her front teeth where her gear kicked in and she finished the task vigorously, up, down, front, back. Thereafter, for a year she brushed morning and night with competent enthusiasm but only when the brush was touched to her teeth by somebody else. Eventually she forgot brushing altogether and the aide or I did it for her.

Her increasing need to be spoon-fed was puzzling. Her grip on a security bar in the bathroom could hardly be broken without her reluctant consent, finger by finger, but her brain would not put a spoon through the evolution that moved food from plate to mouth. She would sit for an hour looking at dinner without interest, unresponsive to guileful urging. Occasionally and unpredictably, just often enough to make us think the idea of feeding herself was there, she applied a spoon to ice cream or applesauce or picked up something bite-size on bread — peanut butter and jelly, hummus, egg salad — for not more than several bites, enough so that it seemed to take the edge off her hunger and no more.

"Would you like some nuts?"

She accepted one with satisfaction, then ignored the bowl-full set on the table beside her. If somebody brought them to her lips she accepted one after another as fast as she could comfortably chew them down.

We tested theories. If she would pick up one chip of cheese on toast, why not, if given time, enough chips to equal a sandwich? If we left her alone with an appetite and a plateful, might she not catch on that it was up to her? Yes, if we allowed an hour or two, and then she would have taken only a few finger-bits.

What if we filled the spoon with Cream of Wheat and left the rest to her? Her invariable response was to dump it; somewhere along the line she had learned a rule that a spoon or fork in her hand was to be returned to the plate and dumped.

Most slippages were not as fast as tooth brushing, most took a few months to be confirmed. Stella continued to feed herself at least a little of certain favorite foods like applesauce and anything chocolate; after a time she did this less often, and finally not at all.

The drill evolved: One of us would sit by with a spoon, and wait for her mouthful to be chewed and swallowed. Then she would accept another. If a helper, wanting to get on with it, filled the spoon too full, Stella shook her head or narrowed her bite. She opened her lips but clenched her teeth. Her jaw trembled, it seemed as though it were trying to open. Suddenly her mouth would spring open, then close before more than a sliver of apricot slipped through to be bitten off, chewed at length, and enjoyed enough to show she would take more if we kept at it.

Unaccountably, then, in the course of a meal her rhythm seemed to change and she would accept whatever was offered without resistance and finish a creditable amount while I counted calories in my head, going for four hundred: goal! The necessary rest was done in sips and snacks. She sipped one or two cans of high-calorie, high-protein diet supplements daily. Her weight fell at no more than the rate of a pound a year. Dr. Loughrand's successor complimented us on that.

She began forgetting for whole meals how to order her mouth to open. Her lips opened, her teeth remained clenched. I learned to wedge my thumb between her teeth. Her mouth might spring open. Sometimes it snapped closed on my thumb. All the while she was trying as hard as we were to find the code that opened the way for food she wanted. As meals went on she tired from the concentration. Her head, naturally inclined forward on account of her osteoporotic curve, dropped farther, blocking ready access to her mouth.

I hated the act of forcing her head up so a spoon could be worked into her mouth. More than other duties that some might find more troubling, it seemed to me that feeding her that way diminished her far beneath her remaining considerable humanity. I became concerned that we had an intractable problem and asked a therapist for guidance. She said it might soon be necessary to feed Stella by tube. It was one of the few times I really felt at the end of my rope. I walked out of her office with wet eyes.

By my measure of "soon" the therapist was wrong. The solution to much of the feeding problem awaited a simple inspiration — instead of dining at the table, we served her in her recliner, angled back just enough to bring her head erect. There is a widespread conviction that lying down during or after meals causes serious digestive problems, but for some people, especially those with forward back curvature, lying back a few degrees can be critically helpful.

We acquired a new doctor of record, Loughrand's successor having retired to a restricted schedule for his own health. I quickly came to like and respect Dr. Milton for the kinds of questions he asked and his close attention to the answers. He had seen Stella once for a full work-up and then again with a digestive problem. Eventually reclining for meals ceased to be effective and I took a puzzle to him: "She seems to have forgotten how to open her mouth. It isn't that she doesn't want to eat. She just can't seem to get the message through to her mouth. She gets her lips parted but the teeth stay shut tight. How can we feed her?"

We had done the obvious by converting her diet to mostly high-calorie liquids, baby foods, and home-blenderings offered through straws, infant sipping cups. We had tried plastic flatware, less menacing than metal in probing for leverage between upper and lower teeth. Portions were small. Time allotted was as much as needed, as often as she was receptive. Stella was not the first difficult feeder Grita and Joan had nursed.

Her face contorted with effort as she sipped small drafts of liquid while we coached, "Wider. Open your teeth." With unlimited persistence and patience Grita and Joan were making the calorie quota, but the day care gave up: "Ate and drank nothing today, sorry to say." We picked up the calorie loss at home with more snacks, longer hours. No strategy really worked. She was eating very little. We were getting behind on liquids. The effort exhausted her. She fell asleep at the table.

This was the puzzle I took to Stella's new doctor. While we talked, he fingered his jaw for a pressure point to spring it.

Obviously it was not something he had had to learn before now. I told him it was just forward of the jaw hinge and painful, to be reserved for emergencies, although repetition might accustom her to open reflexively to the pressure. Anything else?

He said that her esophagus might lose tone, compounding difficult feeding with difficult swallowing.

Those were problems. Were there solutions? Dr. Milton said that if anybody knew it would be nurses. I had already tried the nurse at the Swallowing Clinic, but her expertise began in the mouth, behind the teeth, where we had no access. I had asked our dentist and his assistant: How did they get behind the teeth to clean if the jaw wouldn't open? They had no method. They winged it, lucked it, won some, lost some.

I went to see a nurse on the Alzheimer's floor of a nursing home where there were forty patients in every stage, with every degree of loss. Among them must be recalcitrant feeders. But she too knew only what Grita and Joan and I knew.

She did know one thing she thought I should know. "Sooner or later they refuse food. It is then near the end."

The warning was blunt and somber, from the most experienced observer I could imagine, but she had missed the immediate point. "She isn't refusing. She is trying to open her mouth and isn't succeeding. Once food gets inside her mouth she enjoys it. She enjoys the act of chewing. She enjoys many foods after we fight them between her teeth."

The nurse could not say how we might do any better than we already were.

I talked to everyone and read everything I could find, including a recommended text dug out of the internet by somebody in our daughter's network: *Management of Neurogenic Dysphasia.* Unfortunately, the text began where the Swallowing Clinic's began: behind the teeth. (Nevertheless, it did inform me of ways food could be gotten into the digestive system without passing through the lips. Without intending to, it convinced me that nasogastric tubes would never be installed in my wife or in anybody else for whom I had responsibility. Nor do I detect in myself enough will to live to want it done to me, unless for a day or two in order to get on with a test or other transient procedure.)

One day I noticed in a drugstore a small plastic siphon made for infant feeding. It sucked up a portion of liquid and dispensed it by thumb pressure. It looked like something that could be maneuvered into a cheek pocket to squirt an ounce or two of nutriment.

This little two-dollar device became the backbone of our feeding regimen for liquids and slippy solids, accounting for half the nourishment Stella ingested. I told my children that if I went to a nursing home, to pay more attention to the feeding routine than to anything else — to use it as the key to all the rest of the care — and to be sure that they knew about the baby feeder.

I am sure that thousands of nurses and caregivers know this but nobody told us. I told the Alzheimer's nurse and Dr. Milton. Doctoral treatises have been developed for less. It is likely that I will now find out that it is such common knowledge that it never occurred to anybody that we didn't know it.

EATING and walking were our main concerns. If she ate and walked easily there would have been a kind of normality to her life. I asked the neurologist if anything could be done about her failing ability to walk, even to shuffle. No, it was Alzheimer's.

"There are three kinds of walking. The normal walk with arms swinging. The Parkinson's walk with arms held rigid at the side. The Alzheimer's shuffle." Then, unfortunately, there was no walking.

The neurologist was an affable man not greatly interested in patients; at least not in this particular one. He had seen a television spectacular the night before and wanted to describe it and draw me into a discussion of the romantic life of the star and movies I may have seen him in. As to Stella walking, nothing could be done.

But there was something I figured out. It did not last long, but it was something. One day I urged her on with the *dum-dum-te-dum-dum* of "Stars and Stripes Forever" to take long steps, to lift her knees high. In a moment her foot became unglued from the floor, a knee whipped up and she was marching. She smiled gleefully until after a few steps she lost the rhythm. She couldn't be persuaded just then to try again, but on other days after this initial discovery she would respond to the command, "March!" The neural paths of marching are apparently different from the paths of walking — if the neurologist knew that, he did not share his knowledge.

I was often impressed by how little interest even expert people have about knowledge just around the corner from their specialties. It is equally frustrating to hear them speak of "communicating" as something they do, and how little they seem to understand that nothing happens until information is received. It is hardly likely that what a layman knows is unknown to professionals. A therapist knew about marching; and dancing, too.

To transfer Stella from her recliner to the porch, we grasped wrists and I drew her up. She readily accepted my lead and we took a few dancing steps before resuming her hesitant pace for the last few shuffles to the destination. One of her appearances in her college yearbook was in the gauzy costume of the Dance Club. I was never more than a stolid 4/4 dancer and came into my time during slow tunes, parked in a corner of the floor, bundled with her, rocking side to side. I did better than that in my old age, dancing backward down the hall, gripping her wrists while her feet stammered forward. She liked to go that way much more than with the walker, which steered like a strong-minded Ouija board into chair legs and door frames.

She never got the hang of the walker. I timed her one day walking from the bedroom, down the hall, and across a room to her recliner, a distance of about fifty feet, at a foot a minute, stalling at doorjambs and furniture, nosing along in mouse fractions, before I gave up (she hadn't) short of her destination and moved the walker a half inch from where it had reached under a table and stalled against an obstructing leg. Dancing was better.

CHRISTMAS was at our son's that year. The children asked if I didn't think we should change the usual rotation and have Christmas with Mother in her own home, but I thought it might be the last time she was mobile enough to make a trip and we should do it.

We walked slowly from the car, Stella leaning and half-supported on my arm but doing her share; three steps up to the porch. By the end of the weekend, she could hardly stand unsupported. At the command, "March!" her machinery wanted to start up; in her eyes was evidence of effort being mobilized; she hummed a motoring sound as she often did in the throe of effort. Her foot stirred, but the message did not get through. A son on one side and a son-in-law on the other carried her slumping weight to the car. On the way home, I stopped at the medical supply store and put a wheelchair in the trunk.

So it was that Stella came to need a wheelchair to move more than a few steps, and in a few months she became wheelchair-bound. Being bound so early must be uncommon; I know hundreds of people with Alzheimer's, and only one other became chair-bound when only halfway into the third year. Wheelchairs are expected, but later. None of Stella's doctors suggested it, and I learned too late for it to be even theoretically useful, that such an early disability was, like depression, associated but not necessarily inherent in Alzheimer's. Its differentiated focus in the hippocampus area of the brain may be subject to a medical regime different from Alzheimer's.

Not only is Stella wheelchair-bound, she is unable to move herself around by the handrings that rotate the wheels. Her brain cannot mobilize her hands for that assignment. The exercise therapist who said, "Oh yes, we do that," when I told her about marching could not persuade Stella to do the lesser act necessary to turn the wheels, as the speech therapist had been unable to raise the volume of Stella's voice enough to be heard in the adjoining room when calling for help. Those neural pathways were gone. Where they were is illustrated in the textbook as a Medusa-like tangle of nerve ends and a rubble of dead cells. The alternate locomotion is for the caregiver to push. I unbolted the rings and put them in a closet, and the chair, narrowed by three inches, became miles easier to steer through doors right-angled off the bedroom hall.

Now that I understood getting the chair around narrow corners, I traded down to a smaller model, looking for maximum maneuverability with the minimum loss of comfort. With the addition of a seat cushion filled with high-tech gel, the smallest chair became as comfortable as the biggest and steered readily through the halls and door openings of our ordinary house. It folded to a neat size that slipped into the space behind the driver's seat.

And so we went companionably into the third year. Box-holders met at the post office asked, "Is she still at home with you? Does she know you?" I explained as best I could the world that remained coherent to her: new colors showing in the garden, pictures of houses and table settings in magazines, Christmas cards, Errol Garner or Piatigorsky discs, Fred Astaire reruns. The programs she wanted to stop at when I flipped the stations — never guns or shouting panelists or soap operas, and fewer baseball and basketball games than last year — were about nature, dialogues about books and news, Cosby and Seinfeld comedies of modern manners.

Her eyes kindled for her children and grandchildren and ever fewer friends. When I thought she dozed, the press of osteoporosis bending her chin to her chest, eyes closed, only nominally present, she would suddenly surface with, "I love you, dear," and clasped my hand when I placed it in hers.

I can always generate a conversation — two or three words and attentive eyes — with a question from the past. "Do you remember — ?" The people she had worked with where we had met. Friends from her hometown and schools. Her acknowledgment is immediate and firm. Did she remember our first house? On a March night a chimney fire burned it down, a spectacle for everybody awake late enough at night to see a glow in the sky and come closer to investigate. We had that day brought home armsful of clothes from the cleaners, just in time to be destroyed. We got out in nightclothes and bathrobes, saving nothing but the old Ford backed just in time from the garage under the house. Stella wanted me to remember a little more. She had also saved the kitchen stool, grabbing it on the way out the kitchen door. Yes, she nodded.

We returned early next morning to see one of the neatest fires that had ever taken down a house. The chimney stood as they do after fires, this one a monument to its own malfeasance. We had been in the house only six months, and in the sparse garden of plantings from the fall we looked for the cluster of three rose bushes that had been a house gift from a friend. Where they had been were the holes they had been yanked from. If I didn't have the constitution of an unreconstructed liberal, those three rough holes left in the garden when the last neighbor went home might have been all I wanted to know about human nature.

Did she remember our next house, beyond the suburbs, where they have since leveled the hills and covered the roads and built an airport? It had been a farmer's house before a couple who were good amateur cooks made it a country restaurant, an old ranch bell posted by the road giving it a name and a trademark. The Sunday chicken dinners must not have been attractive enough to bring people that far on an untrafficked road. The real-estate man thought we could make it a house again: a white cottage with a wide lawn, mostly close-cropped weed, contained in one of those loops of old road that look as if they had been going too fast, skittered off, and almost hit the house before recovering and regaining the course.

"Dinner bell," she said.

Where the loop of driveway entered, the cooks had left the dinner bell nested in a fork cut from a locust tree. Local kids, rocketing by at midnight, banged the bell and took off, but not often enough to make us give in and take the bell down. She shook with laughter.

"You're remembering the dinner bell," I said.

Emphatically yes.

"You're remembering the Sunday afternoon Dan and Annie came out to picnic. The summer before Pearl Harbor."

She wanted more names.

"Tom and Duck were there."

And more. It was a word game. Our team was winning. "Barbara ——" and another Tom who was part of Barbara. "Fred ——" and another Anne, who was never Annie, who was part of Fred.

She kept jabbing her finger at me to stay with it until I had it all — the car in the driveway and a man and woman we didn't know getting out, looking around uncertainly, expecting something other than picnickers on the lawn. I approached, and the visitor asked if we were serving dinner.

I explained that it was no longer a restaurant, it had been our home for a year.

"We had dinner here — last month?" He looked to his companion for verification. Maybe two months. At most.

I explained again that it had not been a restaurant for a year. They went away unconvinced. All of this was stored in Stella's head, the visitors going out the driveway, past the dinner bell, the arm of the driver gesturing at it out the window, faulting me for misleading him. She remembered it as well as I did, maybe better.

Her memory did not unpeel in the orderly way it often does after a concussion. We had a friend who was first down the mountain and crashed while we were still tramping into our skis. Unbloody but blank, he seemed to know us but not very well. His brother, a doctor, looked him over carefully and told us to get him into bed in the cabin and keep him warm. Every few hours over three days we asked questions to test his memory as it groped out of the concussion. In the beginning he seemed to remember nothing until we went back twenty-five years — the president after Wilson? As he healed we came forward — after Harding? Mickey Mouse? The stock market crash? Pearl Harbor? The bomb? Television? Lacey's party?

The only question he refused until packing to go home was How many children do you have? Presidents were merely a test, but children were not to be forgotten. Jack's memory turned like calendar pages, one after another in sequence. The further back we go with Stella, the better she is, but it is relative; some pages can be missing in any year.

Periodically the clinic tests her with questions like the one Jack declined. She too is reluctant. Uncomfortable with interrogation she averts her face and looks to me to help her out, but I am not allowed. "Six," she says. I can't sit there and watch her struggle. Why is it important to them? They know her memory is disabled. They are accumulating a research record at an emotional cost — higher for me than for her — I don't want to bear.

"Yes," I interject. "You are including grandchildren. That's okay."

The number is wrong for grandchildren too. The difference between children and grandchildren are indistinct for her but she knows they are hers. I tell the clinic that I don't want to upset their protocol, but if they want Stella to answer questions that are not merely difficult, like numbers, but soul-searching I would like it to be left to me. I will ask her in my own way and let them know.

My method is to pretend that my own memory, which is bad enough, is worse than it is. "I can't remember the name of our friend, the woman who comes and spends a couple of days with you every week. What is her name?"

She surely knows but she cannot say it. When I remember, "Grita!" the quality of her agreement — the quickness, the firmness — are the clues. Multiple-choice tests are okay.

She knows her children and grandchildren. If I ask her to recall unprompted, out of the blue, a name she knows, she can no more do it than recite the state capitals. If I offer a correct name, she recognizes it. If I prompt her with a wrong name she mulls it over, trying to find its place. Sometimes she accepts a name reluctantly, thinking it will humor me. I know when to put it down as denial.

Joking: "Sometimes I forget my own name. What's my name?"

Her reaction is that the question is funny, but she is uneasy that she may be wrong. When I repeat it and seem to really want to know, she has it. "Aaron."

To her, forgetting is not a remarkable experience. She has the concept of what forgetting is and knows it happens to her. Sometimes it frustrates her, she digs at it a little before shaking it off. I expect to be the last name she can get unprompted; she sees me every day.

In my capacity as primary physician, I had not only the major responsibility to choose Stella's doctors and experimental drugs, but also had subordinate and necessary jobs anytime she had a medical incident. There was an early episode at the dinner table in which hoarse and urgent sounds suddenly issued from her; more like exorcism or terminal rattles than anything I had ever heard. She was doubled over so I could see hardly more than her eyes, which were teared with effort, fearful and beseeching. Her eyes also communicated that she trusted that familiar people were working on whatever had seized her.

I punched the 911 button while Grita patted Stella's back as firmly as she dared, in consideration of her fragility. The dispatcher coached me; the squad was on the way.

"Is something lodged in her throat? Can you get a finger in there and make her gag? You know the Heimlich? Get behind her. Lock your fists under her breastbone. Jolt in and up. Elevate her chin. Get your hand under her chin and raise it."

I couldn't get a finger through her set teeth. I didn't dare jolt her with a Heimlich for fear of breaking her back. The unearthly groaning began to ebb when I dragged her chin higher, higher, against the resistant angle of her neck, and the squad pushed in. Soon she was quiet and exhausted.

They guessed her drooping chin had clamped her throat shut. She had been strangling. Her guardians would have to be careful not to let her head fall forward. Keep a pillow under her chin. All agreed that the matter having gone this far, it should be completed with a run to the hospital to let them check her out.

The hospital emergency staff picked up efficiently: history, temperature, blood test, chest X ray. They had her on her back on the gurney, awaiting a decision by a competent authority to assign her a room or send her home and did not notice that osteoporotic curvature craned her head up uncomfortably. By then she was smiling wanly. The primary physician — I — rolled a towel and slid it under her neck. I pulled the blanket up over her naked shoulders. As she had had nothing to drink for hours and the request for water seemed to be wrongly timed to make it happen, I found a machine that sold ginger ale. She sipped it with relish. She had not complained. I was her awareness. I found a second blanket for her when the room temperature dropped.

They decided to keep her overnight. The doctor came in

the morning and said she was okay. I was prepared to check out, but the floor nurse said they would have to wait until the doctor came again to sign the patient out. At seven o'clock in the evening the doctor had not returned. The floor nurse said he had gone home, we would have to wait until morning.

"Oh no," I said. "There's nothing the matter with her. Please get somebody to sign her out."

"It has to be her doctor. He's at home. He'll be back in the morning."

"Call him."

"I can't do that. We don't call him at home."

"Give me his number. I'll call him."

She called him. She explained the problem apologetically. She said things like "Of course" and "I understand" and was about to hang up and convey his rejection with some satisfaction when I asked for the phone. By then an audience of nurses had gathered. I found the doctor not at all difficult to talk to. The doctor asked to speak to the floor nurse again. The patient was soon in the car on the way home. It could have happened as well before lunch or the night before. Of such episodes is the deficit in the national health account compounded.

No matter how many doctors, nurses, and aides Stella would come to need in the passage through Alzheimer's, I knew I would not be a spectator; I would have at least a minor function.

WHAT I could not foresee was that among my virtues as caregiver was what I had previously considered a mild disability — I didn't sleep long. If I put four hours together after midnight I was ready to get up without reluctance and read, garden in season, shovel snow, boot up the word processor, or close my eyes for another restless hour or two. If lost sleep caught up with me later in the day, fifteen minutes in a recliner restored me. (A couple of years later I needed a half hour. Today I can use a half hour morning and many afternoons. If I am in the car, I pull off the road and recline the seat.) It may be genes: my father came home from long, hard days downtown and after dinner napped in his chair, the newspaper slack in his hand. In a few minutes he was ready for a bridge game, a movie, or whatever else my mother had planned for the evening.

The habit of sleep that wakens me ready to go to work at four in the morning more or less coincides with the cycle of Stella's urinary incontinence, so that I am available for duty at useful intervals. I turn on a low light, tell her why I am disturbing her, and raise her enough to draw out the top absorbent mat, leaving the dry undermat in place. I slip out her more personal gauze pad and replace it with another; kiss her on the cheek, tell her I'm done and to go back to sleep. Five minutes. She probably had not really wakened.

In any event, no doctor would do that for her or figure out a better way. Doctors know prescriptions and devices. The doctor said, "No liquid after the evening meal"; but he also said, "Eight glasses of liquid per day." It wasn't easy to make the quota. Stella had forgotten how to part her lips to accept the drinks she very much wanted. It would be up to the caregiver to get it done.

ONE day the director of CenterDay said, as the facilitator at the Alzheimer's Center had a year before, that she was sorry, but she would have to ask me to withdraw Stella. Stella had been in the program for a year, and the reports from the staff had all been good. These were days she never wanted to miss. Her center days were not violated by appointments with dentists, podiatrists, ophthalmologists, beauticians. If she was ready to sleep an extra hour in the morning, as she often was, I had only to say it was a center day, and her eyes widened in readiness. What had happened that made this blessed island in her life no longer habitable?

Nothing sudden. While the encroachment of disability had been by inches, the center now saw a mile of distance between the routine attention other clients required and Stella's need to be fed and toileted and moved always in the wheelchair.

I had not been able to solve the social problem when Stella slipped below the participatory level of her first Alzheimer's group, but this time I saw a glimmer of possibility. The center's problem with Stella was physical. They couldn't lift her and turn her and handle her toileting. They hadn't the hands for individual feeding. Our Alzheimer's office publishes a list of all the day-care facilities in the area, with a rundown of their hours and costs, what they can do and what they can't do: CenterDay cannot handle aggressive people, total incontinence, total wheelchair-bound, total feeding. Some of that included Stella.

What if we hired an aide to be with Stella for the functions she needed?

That would be fine. CenterDay had a list of aides looking for short work weeks. They weren't Gritas, but they were known to be responsible. They could do what was necessary. A bonus was that they also could use their own automobiles to call for Stella in the morning and bring her home in the afternoon, a service forbidden aides provided by agencies.

Being allowed to dispense medication prescribed by a

physician — Stella's pills for osteoporosis, Alz, arthritis — was another bonus of privately employed aides that agency aides below the grade level of "skilled nurse" were not allowed to perform. The more system there is, the more it becomes loaded with prerogatives, the less it focuses on the patient, the more it focuses on itself and its relationship to other systems (no pills, no driving, no work after 6 PM, no lifting, no weekends, no holidays).

Still later a new day program began under the sponsorship of a nursing home a few miles down the road from where we lived, so near that I was bound to look into it. BayEdge Nursing, the primary facility, was a handsome property that a casual traveler might mistake for one of the several resort hotels on the road. Its day program, in a separate, homelike facility built for the purpose, was staffed for everything: incontinence, feeding, a wheelchair van for transport.

Stella had so enjoyed CenterDay that I went about the transfer tentatively, prepared to call it off if she did not adjust well to the change. For continuity's sake, we kept a day a week at CenterDay. I need not have been concerned. From the first morning the new program at BayEdge worked for her as well as the old at CenterDay.

Some people with Alzheimer's are in a perpetual state of unrest and dissatisfaction. Stella accepted with equanimity much that she would have balked at before. Somebody else had to notice for her that she was sitting in a draft or too long in a stiff chair. One day care was much the same as another: pleasant company, things going on, lunch, snacks. CenterDay was scheduled out and a third day added at BayEdge.

Stella never asked what had happened to those nice people she had spent a year with at CenterDay. I try to visualize her inner experience of putting aside the year at the center as she had put aside a life experience when her sister died. I say *put aside* and avoid *forgotten* because the memory remains latent; it is the recall that does not happen unless prompted. Is her experience like the intense but momentary attention you and I give newspaper stories of the tragedies and lottery winnings of people who go out of our lives as we turn the page? We remember the incidents only when recall is clued to us, as Stella remembers when she is asked. Her sister (or mine, who became her closest friend) and the year at the center are drained of emotion for her, as if the color has been washed out and only identifiable shapes remain.

Her life is lived in the present. Those of us who are here are here. Others are filed. My sister has not been mentioned since she died two years ago. "Stell," I ask, "Do you remember when we went to Vermont with Eve to see the fall colors in the mountains?" She remembered enough. "I hadn't made a reservation at an inn or motel. It was the middle of the foliage season. Everybody was in Vermont to see the color and we didn't have a room to stay in. Do you remember that? My sister Eve was with us." She had more. "We got the last room in the worst motel in Vermont. It wasn't a very big room. They used it as a storage room and opened it up for us. They put a cot in for Eve. She had to crawl over us if she wanted to get in or out of bed. Eve said she would never go anywhere with us again."

She enjoyed that. "Eve. Yes."

READING *Elegy for Iris*, a book John Bayley wrote about his life as caregiver to his wife, Iris Murdoch, as she fell into Alzheimer's, I was struck by the similarities between Bayley's emotional life and mine and the differences between the Alzheimer's experiences of the two women.

Iris Murdoch was aware of herself slipping away as Stella was not. Bayley feared that his wife would wander from the house toward risk; I think of wandering as a lost privilege. Scores of disabilities emerge when you can't get to your feet and walk to the garden or bathroom, walk the aisles of a store, follow the hostess to a table in a restaurant, take the few stairs to the bedrooms in your children's houses.

I readily understand the complex devotion Bayley had for Murdoch, but even his most empathetic friends, and certainly distant readers of his book, may speculate, Didn't the relationship become a duty, a habit, a chore? Couldn't he afford better alternatives? How could he not prefer a night at the theater with old friends to sitting alone reading while she slept in another room? Literary people have excessive imaginations; did Bayley talk himself into a mood of pseudo-gallantry?

I know that isn't it at all, no part of it. He loved the girl. That is what love is for him. It was not a duty but a grace to be a presence to her as she was to him; to be all the memory she had; to have a hand to offer that might not be as skilled as a nurse's but one she trusted, as hers was the one he knew in every freckle, vein, and sinew and liked to have rest in his. Bayley wrote his memoir in the second year of Alzheimer's, then near his wife's last days. In my fifth, I understand that Bayley still had the girl he fell in love with when she rode by him on a bicycle. I fell in love with Stella in a department store when she walked by, manila folder in hand, on a mission from the personnel department to the buyer of housewares. Like Bayley, I led my love to a riverbank, ours the mountain stream whose headwater ran under what became the famous house Fallingwater. Like Bayley, I never got over it.

8

PAYING THE BILL

WE COULD USUALLY TELL if a new girl in the store
worked in personnel: she was a visual bulletin from the personnel manager that this is what the store ought to look like.

The new girl had the personnel imprint: she was good-
looking in the way men's tie department girls — who may
have been even better-looking — weren't. She looked like a
women's college grad. Standing still, she looked like she knew

where she was going; was going *to,* not waiting *for.* Of course, men's tie girls didn't walk around the store carrying papers.

The new girl had business with the same buyers and merchandise managers I did. It wasn't long before we knew each other's names and what we did. She was on my mind, but I couldn't afford even a movie date. I thought I might have to ask her if she had ever been to the zoo.

I worked for a vice president and was paid mostly with the honor of having any kind of job in 1938 and a few perks such as the use of his tennis court, freedom to write headlines like "The British Stamp on the U.S. Male," and tickets that went with his obligation to subscribe for almost anything in the arts. One day soon after I set possessive eyes on Stella he dropped two concert tickets on my desk.

I didn't care much for classical music, but it might be better than the zoo to get us together. I went across the floor to the high counter that marked off the personnel bullpen, out of my territory; they worked for a different vice president. I pointed to Stella. She pivoted on the chair, knees locked under a trim gray skirt, which said to me at a glance that she had been raised to stay buttoned-up. She had a walker's strong ankles, she wasn't floppy inside her blouse. She came to the counter looking, I thought hopefully, a little more friendly than merely polite.

"Stella. I have two tickets for the symphony next Wednesday night. How about going with me? I'll pick you up. Where do you live?"

"Could you slow down?"

I had not before seen her eye to eye. They were hazel, her complexion fair. It was July and she hadn't tanned at all, would never tan. I liked it that she wasn't too sophisticated to struggle for an answer while she thought about whether this was the way a date should happen. "Wednesday? The symphony?" Her rather long, narrow Spanish face inched toward a wonderfully open smile. I didn't know then that she was a cellist and almost anybody who showed symphony tickets and had some credentials of acquaintanceship could probably get the date.

A week or two later my vice president won a wrangle with her vice president. For a reason I didn't understand then and don't understand today, my vice president wanted control of sales training. Training employees of retail stores to sell is the kind of department I would want to divest. He had no idea what to do with the victory and put me in charge, and as I knew even less he committed to get me anybody I wanted from the other vice president's side to be my assistant and educate me. They had people over there who had gone to graduate schools of retailing, they had people who had worked for Marshall Field, they had —

"Stella Marcum," I said.

We married three months later, secretly because it was against policy for a married couple to work in the same department. Before anybody could denounce us, we resigned to take our talents elsewhere. My vice president offered Stella a promotion to another department if we would reconsider, but we knew what we wanted to do. Stella was going to teach music in a private school. Marriage had broadened my vision; I had second thoughts about making my career where I had begun as a stock boy at a wage that could hardly increase fast enough to keep me more than minimally afloat.

Many years later, after the war and children and after we had had all the careers we wanted, Stella and I moved to Cape Cod and opened a not very serious store to sell the kinds of things we had liked when we saw them on their native grounds: Portuguese and Dutch tiles, Mexican embroidered shirts, Thai brasses, Japanese woodcuts, fat candles that curled like a Dutch girl's bob, whittled wooden toys. It seemed more like recreation than work. We were together and summer jobs were built-in for the children. Soon we caught on well enough to need staff, and, as Stella was experienced at it, I was glad to cede her the hiring.

"I can eliminate half of the applicants by the way they walk across the floor," she said. People who hire always have methods, standards, prejudices to reduce quantities to convenient numbers. Must have a college degree. Must have a masters. Must look like country club. Must be over five-foot-four. Must walk purposefully.

"That's a good system," I said. "You probably don't lose more than half the best candidates that way."

"If you don't like the staff, you can always fire me and hire them yourself."

I always liked the staff.

We had that career, and another after that. When we arrived at Alzheimer's I guessed, without knowing very much about it, that Medicare and its supplement would pick up the main cost, as it had trained us to expect in our other illnesses and injuries; and whatever they didn't pick up we could afford.

Medicare and our supplemental insurance did, in fact, pick up not a part but all the costs to establish the diagnosis: the visits to Drs. Loughrand, Harrison, and Geerey; blood tests and brain scan. But Medicare's part in Alzheimer's ended there. It took me not months but years to penetrate the armor of home-care agencies and Medicare in order to get to the core ruling: Inasmuch as it was Alzheimer's, Medicare did not cover anything after the diagnosis — not a dime's worth, nothing. Any investment in time and postage to pin down that fact and its illogical ramifications was simply wasted.

Medicare covered medical costs that were the consequence of Alzheimer's — breaks from falls, pneumonia, bed sores — but none of the costs of Alzheimer's care that prevented such costly consequences.

CONSIDERING the large role financing the illness plays in the life of most people with Alzheimer's, the literature has remarkably little to say about it. Excepting perfunctory suggestions to consult my lawyer or financial adviser, how the condition was to be paid for was excluded from every book about Alz I picked up to prepare myself to be Stella's caregiver. That I had either lawyer or adviser, that if I had them the lawyer would know much more than real-estate law, the financial adviser much more than his portfolio of funds and theories of assets allocation, were assumptions that should be examined by every writer before meddling in the lives of caregivers.

IT is difficult to put on an acceptable face to write about your own financial circumstances; unless, that is, you are poor, or disadvantaged in some other way, which we are not, except for Stella's illness. Readers are biased in favor of characters who can't pay their bills. Reading about hardscrabble lives stirs emotions of empathy and admiration for those who endure, best wishes in the struggle up (but not, we should admit, a feeling of envy). When life became for me writing-about-life, the romantic personality of hard economic luck was not available.

Nor was its opposite. In prosperous characters we look for the entertaining spectacle of excess — big houses, private airplanes, dinners at the Ritz — and the likelihood of a fall from grace. I don't doubt that some readers anticipate with unadmitted satisfaction the episode in which a just or unfathomable fate overtakes the husband and he is forced to admit that the care of his wife has broken him as it breaks hundreds of thousands of others. Life is long but I am near its end and I don't foresee that kind of ruin.

In the character of a caregiver in a book, I may be doubly miscast: not only am I not being ground down to desperation by the financial burden, but I can't take more than one martini without getting sick, so, like Stella, I am a one-drink drinker. Like running out of money, being driven to drink by stressful circumstances — or by genes or bravado — is more interesting in literature than in real life.

Above all, I want to avoid implying that my situation is in any sense extreme. Everybody knows far worse cases, if not in life, then on television or in the papers. My situation doesn't compare favorably with daughters who give up good jobs for dead ends in order to get home for a few minutes every day to give medication or change an incontinent's clothes. This entire special pleading for the Alzheimer's aged — one Alzheimer's aged — has to be read in the light of millions, hundreds of impoverished millions, in shot-up, bombed-out, raped nations, suffering from so many disasters that trail off far beyond our Adult Deficit Attention Spans.

Nevertheless, Stella is in her fifth year of Alzheimer's, wheelchair-bound, barely able to communicate, and I am her caregiver, sharing the experience of it with you, hoping it enlarges your understanding of what Alzheimer's can be, as the disease will almost certainly come into your life if you live long enough. Here are a few snapshots, enough to let you compare our circumstances with yours: When we married,

Stella and I together earned less than eighty dollars a week, not a bad amount when an almost-new $450 Ford and a mint-new $5500 house were affordable on a $4000 income. We budgeted mortgage, utilities, insurance, and car in a checking account that sometimes missed the required minimum balance, then $50. Household expenses were budgeted in the three pockets of a spare bathrobe: one pocket food and other ordinaries, one pocket available to either of us at will if anything was in it, one pocket tithe. I admit to half-tithes until I came home after the war, got down to business, and gave up bathrobe budgeting.

Certainly we are in a well-off percentile, but families with wealth more confirmed than ours are able to tithe away half and more of income with no more inconvenience than we pledge our tenth. Much of life is luck. Longevity seems to be in our genes; after sixty years of marriage, we have outlived mortgages and needy relatives. I got over the idea that I especially deserved success when my insightfully chosen stocks came out no better than even with the investments of a chimpanzee that threw darts at the financial page.

Our children are middle-class as we are. Educations for three generations have been accomplished without scholarships of need, which took only a part-time job for me in the 1930s; a workable fraction of a young family's income when our children went to college in the 1960s; and is still manageable when degrees for grandchildren rear up as nondeductible monsters with an appetite for entire family incomes. Our car is an unsophisticated nameplate going on five years old. We live in a house that isn't worth as much as the view; the yearly tax is less than three thousand dollars. A person of means might want to tear it down and build something with higher ceilings; we are not that tall.

In any event, I arrived at the role of caregiver confident that I could handle the economic cost. I did not look to Medicare for a very large part of it. Had anyone told me about Medicare and Alzheimer's I would not have bothered to look to that resource for any part at all, which would have been the right amount.

This is mostly a Medicare war story because Alzheimer's is a disease of the generation that acquired its health-care coverage before the era of HMOS. Take it as a warning to look for similar terrain in your own coverage.

How Medicare positions itself in order not to cover Alzheimer's is of considerable importance, inasmuch as the same rule that eliminates thousands who can afford the loss draws blood from millions who need it and thought their Medicare would in due time cover.

Aides, not hospitals or doctors, are our main expense. They began with the two days Grita could spare for us. As Stella's condition worsened, other aides came in. The agency whose aides covered some of the hours told me that Medicare's standard practice was to allow one-and-a-half hours every morning to get Stella up, toileted, bathed, and breakfasted, and another one-and-a-half hours for end of the day tasks.

I thought reimbursement of twenty-one hours out of what had become fifty aide hours (and later, sixty — and later still, ninety) was minimal but if that was the established schedule I did not challenge it. At an average cost of $15 an hour, Medicare would relieve me of $16,000 of annual aides cost that passed $40,000 before the second year in Alz ended, $50,000 before the end of the third. And the cost rises.

There was a catch. The manager of the licensed home-care agency, the voice of Medicare, said that if Stella went to a day care that was not medically certified, Medicare would pay none of the aide costs. Stella was then going to CenterDay, a facility sponsored by our Council on Aging, but it was not certified as a place where medical services could be arranged. Its uncertified status nullified any home-care coverage Stella might otherwise be due, I was warned.

I thought Medicare misunderstood: I was not asking for coverage of CenterDay or the private aide they required Stella to have. My request was for aides who came to our home in the morning and late afternoon, before and after Stella was at CenterDay. These were services Stella had to have in order to get out of bed, to be bathed, fed, and made ready for the start and finish of the day.

No matter. Medicare did not pay bills for aides if the patient went to a day care that was not medically approved.

That was the first I heard about there being two kinds of day-care services. Until BayEdge opened, no medically approved day program went on anywhere near us, and I would not even think about withdrawing Stella from CenterDay, which had become such a satisfying part of her life. She had limited medical needs but very much needed the social life of a group. Dr. Loughrand had prescribed it, and far more authorities agreed on the value of socializing than agreed on the medical value of tacrine, then the only FDA-approved drug. I thought the ruling idiotic, but there are many idiotic things in life and it was not my first adult experience of Alice in Wonderland. I accepted the rules.

When medically certified BayEdge opened and Stella fitted in well there, I went back to the agency and reported that we were now qualified for twenty-one hours of home aide time per week.

Well no, the scheduler said, I must have misunderstood. Stella would have to go to BayEdge for medical treatment, and as she did not go there for that reason, but only for the social program (they made it sound like a round of parties) her homebound status would be canceled. If she left home for day program, obviously she was not homebound.

It did not avail that she was wheelchair-bound both at home and at BayEdge and was transported back and forth in a wheelchair van. Medicare's point was that she went out; how could she be homebound if she went out? Reduced to this Zen dilemma, Medicare was an authentic Catch 22 when compared to the original that had been merely a device of comic literature.

I argued that her disability had an identified, certified existence independent of attendance at any day care. How were the necessities of morning and evening care contaminated by the program at BayEdge? How were the four days of the week she did not go there contaminated by the three days she went? How did whatever she did at day care invalidate the certification of four doctors, as well as visiting nurses and therapists, that she was unable to walk or even stand alone while she did it?

If the point was to challenge the applicant's disability, there were many better ways than the rude rule of thumb of day-care attendance. If Medicare was frightened that being homebound might be one more billion-dollar fraud the agency would be hauled before a congressional committee to account for, it could order an examination by a doctor — by a committee of doctors — of its choice at my expense. And anyhow, I urged, forget BayEdge. BayEdge was a red herring. We were not asking for coverage for Stella's BayEdge time. BayEdge was our own uncontested expense from the moment Stella's morning aide ushered her to the van to the moment her evening aide met her at home. The one-and-a-half hour coverage segments we applied for were for other times and other days, for amounts established by experience in the care professions, including Medicare, for the disabling stages of diabetes, stroke, arthritis, and so on. If you had one of those diseases and were disabled to the degree Stella was, Medicare covered, as it covered bedsores, pneumonia, and broken arms.

The answers I received did not address logic. They cited regulations. Regulations were facts of nature. They did not need to be justified anymore than the ocean or a tree or a stone had to be justified. They were there. The regulation stated that if you went out for whatever reason, you were not housebound, and if you were not housebound you did not qualify for aide support.

I was presented with other curious questions, as if to make sure that ordinary standards of reason would not avail. Did she *participate* in the program when she was at BayEdge? On the days she happened to need certified medical services (the two days she had needed a cough medicine administered at noon; the one day every several weeks when she had her toenails cut, not a cosmetic but a medical service restricted to podiatrists by law in our state) — on those days did she stay the whole day or was she brought home promptly after her toenails were cut? Did she stay there after the teaspoon of prescription cough syrup?

I did not see what interest of medical or public policy was served by requiring Stella to come home after she took a pill, or what crime she had committed for which Medicare wanted to confine her to quarters every day. Wasn't it enough that in her twenty-four-hour days she could do nothing unaided — *nothing* — except involuntary functions? The home-care agency shifted ground again. The real bottom line was that Medicare did not cover any condition deemed incurable. Diabetes, stroke, arthritis and so on were curable. Alzheimer's was not. I must have misunderstood that transferring her to a medically approved agency had any effect on her membership in the forbidden society of the incurable.

It didn't look like a bottom line to me. What about hospice? Wasn't a hospice patient by definition not curable? Didn't Medicare cover hospice? Didn't Medicare pay hospital bills for any number of hospital patients classified as terminal? Didn't we both know cases — heart disease, kidney, cancer — no more curable than Stella that received daily home care?

Agreed, the agency said, but there was an even realer bottom line under the real bottom line: Medicare simply did not cover the incurable disease that was Alzheimer's. Period. It was time to give up on the locals and go higher. I wrote to Medicare's master, the Department of Health and Human Services.

From correspondences with the IRS I expected that before anything happened in any bureaucracy a follow-up letter would be needed and, eventually, maybe a request to my congressman to look into it. The public gets answers in time, whenever their inquiries clear the process. To expedite congressional inquiries, higher-grade-level staff is assigned.

Medicare is especially likely to answer the senior senator from Massachusetts or his legislative assistants promptly — Medicare legislation has Ted Kennedy's name on it. There might not be any Medicare at all, only the standing shell, if the senior senator from Massachusetts did not shore it up. It may seem an enormous waste of energy and talent for a United States Senator to act as a mail facilitator, but that is the system. Nobody knows why God put an appendix in the lower right quadrant of the belly, but it's there.

Expect that the answer jacked out of Health and Human Services by the senator will not quite answer your question. Instead, the corporate style answers questions you have not asked. A look of earnestness and accommodation screens the fact that your question has been avoided:

> First, Mr. Alterra [the Government wrote, referring to my letter to the senator], your letter states that you were informed that Medicare does not provide coverage for the treatment of Alzheimer's disease. That is not correct. The Medicare coverage guidelines specify that the need for skilled nursing care must be based on the condition rather than the diagnosis. To qualify for the Medicare home health benefit, the law requires that a Medicare beneficiary be confined to the home, under the care of a physician, receiving services under a plan of care established and periodically reviewed by a physician, be in need of skilled nursing care on an intermittent basis.

Fine. Stella was Loughrand's patient. He examined her. Her disability was total. He affirmed that she needed coverage twenty-four hours a day. He saw her periodically. He got reports from visiting nurses. The skilled nursing provision was taken care of in the convention that existed locally with Medicare's knowledge (and, I had to assume, approval) that services performed by aides were reviewed for an hour or so every month by an RN for her agency's records and passed on to the doctor for his records. Anomalies of the patient's health not already taken to the physician by the caregiver were included in the RN's report. Seeing the system at work, an observer might conclude that the operationally significant part of it was the paper trail laid down to satisfy the regulations.

> Second, the overriding principle in the definition of homebound is that there must be a normal inability to

leave the home and leaving the home requires a considerable and taxing effort.

Again, fine. In detail, Stella's disability was more profound
and extensive than the definition, but if the definition was
good enough for Medicare it was good enough for us. It was
commonsensical, brief and direct, and it was overriding.

Third, if Stella qualified as homebound "Medicare covered either part-time or intermittent home health
aide services and skilled nursing care . . . any number
of days per week as long as they are furnished (combined) less than eight hours of each day and 35 or
fewer hours per week." Additional authorization(s)
could be had for "up to 56 hours per week of daily services as long as the need for these services is for a fi-
nite period of time."

In sum, it appeared that Stella was entitled not only to coverage, but to more than the $315 per week we had asked for,
and the coverage was for skilled nursing care. Our local agencies charged $32 per hour for nurses. If aides instead of nurses
were acceptable to Medicare, as they were to us, the cost
would be half as much, a bargain for Medicare. Our inquiry
had clearly stated that it was on behalf of an Alzheimer's patient. Nothing in the government's response mentioned an ex-
clusion of cases classified as incurable.

But we were at point four, and here was planted the land
mine to blow up everything that had gone before. Medicare
did not even have to get to the simple rock bottom that there
was nothing for Alzheimer's.

If a patient leaves home on a regular basis to attend day care, which does not have a medical purpose, the patient would not meet the homebound requirement and, therefore, would not be eligible for services under the Medicare home health benefit.

The conflict between point two, the simple definition of homebound, and point four, the condition that vetoed it, was clear: two gave, four took away. Taking away prevailed.

Nothing was said about incurable. Incurable was verboten. Alzheimer's was verboten, a word that could be uttered only if attributed to me.

Several levels of appeal were listed for me: reconsideration, hearing before an administrative law judge, department Appeals Board review, and u.s. District Court. One of these venues might see the contradiction between Medicare's own description of what it meant to be homebound and the trivial reasons Medicare had devised to defeat the benefit.

Another level of appeal, the demand letter, was not mentioned. We were in Alzheimer's for years before I heard about demand letters. No home-care agency or Medicare literature mentioned it. No agency scheduler, when advising me that Stella was ineligible for coverage, suggested that I send a demand letter. It wasn't in any published Patient's Bill of Rights. No correspondent from Health and Human Services called it to my attention during our leisurely wrangle about qualifying Stella.

A demand letter is a kind of street knowledge. I heard it mentioned in a caregivers group. When I asked Medicare about it, I got an "oh yeah we got that" answer as if it was last year's style. Perhaps it was what was contemplated as "Reconsideration." Terminologies everywhere have lives of their own.

A demand letter is one that a client asks his home-care

agency to send to Medicare requesting reconsideration of a rejected claim. A client has the right to make the demand. The agency has the duty to take it up with Medicare.

My petition to the agency to make the demand on Medicare reviewed the history of rejections and rested on the contradiction between paragraphs two and four and the function of overriding — their word of choice, not mine.

The law must have been written to benefit the handicapped, not to find a way not to. Nobody could possibly contest Stella's handicap under Medicare's definition of homebound, and if the condition was overriding, what was it meant to override if not such nigglings as what she did at day care and how long she did it?

I don't know how the agency presented the case to Medicare, but the response was terse and negative.

I would have abandoned the claim had I not come upon a magazine article written by our congressman. Embedded in it was a letter from a constituent with Alzheimer's stating his gratitude for the home care Medicare provided him every morning and evening. Home care!! Twice a day! For many many months! For Alzheimer's! Exactly the coverage denied Stella! And for an Alzheimer's patient still possessed of enough faculty to write this explicit, coherent letter!

My flagging interest perked up. I asked the congressman's office people if they could find out in what way that model case differed from Stella's. We seemed to match it or beat it on all fours. The staff obliged but the department's return letter did not respond to the question. Instead of stating what, if anything, in Stella's history did not match an apparently model case, Health and Human Services (and its paymaster, Health Care Financing Administration) patiently stated what its rules were. I pointed out this discrepancy to the congressional office and asked it to try again for a specific answer to the specific question. They did that.

The second reply was as unresponsive as the first.

A legislative office, getting a copy of the letter from government bureaucrat to constituent, does not pay close attention to the contents. The mail facilitator's job is to facilitate mail. If the voter isn't satisfied with the content, he should grind out another letter. I gained an understanding of how the discovery process in a lawsuit could go on for years. No more letters, I resolved, the bureaucrats have an infinite supply of nonsense. They beat me. I never did find out why the Alz case cited by the congressman got a benefit my wife was denied.

At 3:30 the van trundles down the driveway and Henry honks to get me out of wherever I am in the house. The side door opens and cantilevers the elevator platform. While Henry unhooks Stella from the floor buckles I look in the front door and exchange greetings with four other BayEdge regulars on their way home. Stella's is the only wheelchair. Henry wheels her out on the elevator and as she descends I scrub her legs and take her hands and then we are eye to eye. Her face, hooded under the brim of a country denim hat, has been tensed in ritual concern about coming down for the landing. When she touches down, her grin reaffirms the gestures of greeting that have just passed between us. "Was it a good day?"

"Good day."

Not once has it been anything less. She has only to give this up in order to be classified as homebound, from which condition all benefits flow.

Well, not quite. They will come back to square one: Her condition is chronic. They know it is chronic because she has Alzheimer's. It isn't that they don't cover Alzheimer's. It's *chronic* they don't cover. They would cover Alzheimer's if it wasn't chronic. It is an evenhanded policy: rich and poor alike are privileged to sleep under bridges.

ADVERSARIAL relationships with large, remotely centered organizations — governments, insurance companies, stockbrokers, hospitals, automobile manufacturers, newspapers, and so on — don't often succeed without the intervention of lawyers. Lawyers, unless their interest is captured by some appealing peculiarity of a case, can't afford more than the courtesy of a letterhead and a paragraph of basic text for small cases that aren't bundled into something larger, like a practice in workman's compensation, asbestos poisoning, stockholder advocacy, tobacco smoke. Lawyers especially can't afford to be drawn into the body of regulations, regulatory interpretations, and administrative whims by which Medicare is governed.

I heard a legal-aid lawyer speak at a meeting and thought she knew what she was talking about. She invited anybody in the audience who had a problem to get in touch with her at her office. Nominally a service reserved for the Medicaid population, radically underfunded for their mission, legal service corporation lawyers often are approachable by others. They are likely to be well informed about Medicare because so many of their regular constituents have problems with medical services. (Congress tries continually to put legal services out of business by taking away budgets but, as in all such matters, the senior senator from Massachusetts must first be got out of the way.)

I took my demand letter correspondence to her. She looked it over, nodding her head. She had been through this before. Was it worthwhile to carry the case higher, through the four-stage chain of appeals? "It won't get you covered."

Why was that?

"Because it's Alzheimer's. They'll ignore 'overriding.' It's a loose word in the correspondence. It's what a lower level executive, trying to make sense, came up with. In the end, they still won't say Alzheimer's — they'll say chronic; it's chronic. They don't cover chronic, any chronic. Chronic is different from terminal. Chronic is predicted from the front end. Terminal is confirmed at the back end. They'll concede any point but chronic, by which they mean Alzheimer's. They'll give you reasons. Your wife isn't homebound because she goes to day care. If she doesn't go to day care it's still chronic. You can get short runs of coverage, a few days at a time, for bedsores, a bad cold, long toenails, anything your doctor wants a skilled nurse to take a particular look at."

"Skilled nurse" is another ambiguity. Skilled in what? My wife's aides are skilled in the care of a wholly disabled person. We have had registered nurses who couldn't lift her from a chair. Why is the government committed to skilled nurses and nursing homes? They cost twice as much, although, if the patient is on Medicaid, it's a government not a personal expense. An uncounted number of patients would not put the government to the expense of Medicaid if Medicare shared the cost of a few hours of precisely metered aides at the patient's home.

"On the scale of what your wife needs for a year or two or more, forget Medicare. It ain't gonna happen."

The irony in all this was that I thought from the beginning of my experience with Medicare that there should be a means test for all benefits, and that Stella and I should fail it by reason of having a sufficient income. Claims like ours should be rejected, but not by a mindless regulation that traps the deserving with the undeserving which included us.

9

I WANT TO GO HOME

THE NEW YEAR BEGAN WITH a fax from my daughter-in-law at her desk in the hospital. An article in the British medical journal *Lancet* confirms with research what others have guessed: a magnetic resonance instrument can be used to see the site of memory in the living brain. Shrinkage of the entorhinal cortex can be measured. Shrinkage means loss. I think immediately to make a call to a prophet whom I had not talked to in three years, Ina Krillman. I recalled myself to her.

"I want to remind you of a conversation we had. You probably had the same conversation with others. You said you were sure Alzheimer's was present long before it was diagnosed — not months, but years before — and that I should get my wife on medication as quickly as possible. You were a prophet. I'm calling to honor you."

"I wasn't the only one. I thought there was a lot in the theory that Alzheimer's begins in the genes but research seems not to have confirmed it in most cases. What have you got?"

I read key paragraphs to her. "They can measure loss in the very young, in children. It can be a key predictor of Alzheimer's." The armory of drugs was increasing rapidly. Here was the site at which their effect could be measured.

"There is a lot of movement in the field." She changed the subject. "How is your wife — Stella? She was at home with you when we last talked. What can you tell me?"

"She is at home, wheelchair-bound, and her speech is about gone, but she is in good health. She sleeps a lot but is never depressed."

"There are some blessings. She had a delightful and ready smile, I remember. I had to sign my father into a nursing home a few months ago. I couldn't manage any longer. Alzheimer's at ninety, you know."

"Has he adjusted all right?"

"Mostly, I guess. When I see him he places his frail old hand in mine and looks me in the eye and says he wants to go home. It tears me apart. What can I do."

When I think of nursing homes, which is often, as I am in and out of them for caregiver meetings, it seems to me the most wrenching words a caregiver can hear must be, "I want to go home."

GRITA's day that had begun in the morning at eight had ended, leaving Stella and me alone on the porch, having a quiet time together after supper. I kept Stella up on what was going on. I told her where the sun was and that Keiley's cat was waiting for a bird to take a late bath in the blue dish. I hollered to the cat to get out of there. I told her how tree shadows from the southerly ridge put the garden on the evening side of afternoon. I described painterly light. Picked out against darkened foliage and made luminous as if lighted from within were daylilies and roses and all those African and Asian flowers I knew only as daisies (except for the Shasta, our own). I said some of the clumps were crowded, I'd have to dig and separate in the fall. I talked.

Stella hardly noticed. Her chin rested on her chest. Her eyes were closed but I knew she was not sleeping. "Yes," she murmured and "I think so" if I seemed to press for a response.

The last day-sailer came off the bay in a racket of tacks, milking the air for enough power to move the boat through the narrows toward the anchorage. "He's a good sailor." He waved. I waved. I didn't know him in the binoculars. He might know me. We had been a navigation mark for thirty-five years. "He isn't getting more than ten feet on a tack. He'll have to change twenty or thirty times, back and forth, back and forth. That's what I call patience. Wouldn't you say 'There goes a really patient man?'"

"I think so."

I didn't know how much she retained of what went on around her. I assumed it was a lot more than I could be sure of.

That afternoon she had looked at me with such steadiness and penetration that I felt a return in kind was in order. Our gazes locked without wavering until she said unexpectedly, "What do you think you're doing?"

She seldom had more than one or two words. If more dribbled out they were likely to be unintelligible.

I said, "I am looking at you and you are looking at me. I don't know about you, but I like what I see."

She held my eyes for another few seconds and broke into a look of gaiety. "Good answer," she said.

We were still tacking through chocolate pudding. "Another spoonful?"

She tried to muster the acts necessary to open her mouth. Her lips quivered and separated but her teeth remained tight. I thumbed her chin, I probed with the spoon until they opened enough. I have ten times the effortless patience now than I had when impatience was effortless.

We finished dessert. I finished the saga of the good sailor who, nevertheless, had hung up once on the bank and had to get out and shove off. Stella had not opened her eyes. She had said "Yes" and "I think so" when I said how good a sailor he was. For a few quiet minutes I thought she was going to nap. Then the second long, unexpected statement of the day — firmly spoken, disconcerting, "I want to go home."

Nothing had been said that might lead to it. She had not seemed pensive or introspective.

"We *are* home." Treading water — maybe she thought we were at a restaurant. In a light, orienting voice, I elaborated that we lived here; we ate here; we slept here. That's what home was. Home had been here for thirty-five years.

Fewer words mean many more things: "I" consistently means herself, but "you" may be "you" or "they," somebody at day care, a character on the screen, somebody remembered, anybody. "Home" could be another place, another room, a location in another time. It could mean inside the house, anywhere she is not. Images that go with such words seem to be specific in her mind but fade quickly; Roman candles, cards opened in a game of solitaire for which there is no sequence.

I did not suspect an unhealed wound in her memory. Usually I can be sure that nothing as psychoanalytic or novelistic as angst or nostalgia is troubling her. She may confuse which rooms are in this house and which in that, but she is not longing for anything of the past, she is thinking only of a place elsewhere that occurs to her. A room in her parents' house may have drifted to her in an odor or a musical phrase. If I didn't respond as she wished, she would hardly be disappointed. The card would simply go back in her deck, perhaps never again to be played.

"Stay with that a minute" has gone from our conversation. She cannot stay with a subject; she cannot go through layers of possibilities. When I don't get what she has in mind, I can displace it, apparently to her satisfaction, simply by suggesting something we can deal with in common. My part was to try her with a few questions until I proposed something that displaced what had been in her mind with something as satisfactory. Was she talking about the house she had been in when she was a little girl? No. The house in the town we had lived in before this? She looked a little doubtful.

Did she want to move from the porch to her recliner? She said, "Yes." If it was not what she had meant, it was what she had come to mean as the moment moved on.

I don't encourage you to think that words missing their intended destination go underground, are suppressed, should be diligently quizzed out, exposed for the sake of her emotional well-being. The patient's rights man may believe that it is her right not only to be heard but also to be understood, and that her wishes that can be identified should prevail. I think that is a flight of fancy sustained only by the words that say it. The most diligent inquiry may gain her agreement to something she had not thought of and may have little real interest for her. If she assents when I ask if she is thinking of the house she grew up in, shall we pack and make the trip? What needs to be found out is what she can live with comfortably. That's what I want to know on her behalf. She can't always say it. She can't hold options in her mind.

What is absent is not quite real. She never asks for ice cream but is always glad to have it. If she never has it again, she won't ask, "What happened to ice cream?"

Homes, ice cream, people come and go, little valued in memory. Presence is what counts. You can understand with what hesitation I say it would not be traumatic for her to lose a child or a grandchild, hard as it is to believe when you see her light up when they come to see her. If I disappear, she will not have difficulty getting used to my absence. I keep coming back to that astonishing idea: If I am no longer present, it will not take Stella long to get used to it.

NAME the possibilities: heart, kidney, cancer, a heel caught on a stair, a truck crossing the median strip . . . In an odd way it is comforting to know that if I were to go into a hospital and not come out, she would not be as affected as I would be to lose her. If others held open for a while the possibility that my absence was temporary and not press on her the finality and solemnity of death, I am sure she would not sense the extension of time toward infinity. Any loss she felt would not be as deep as sorrow. The capacity for sorrow is something she has lost.

She was not moved by the death of her sister when I received the phone call from her companion. Their sisterly relationship had been close and confiding. They were each other's only sibling and Diane had no children of her own.

"Diane died this morning."

It did catch her a little. "That's too bad."

"She was comfortable. I'll make a few calls and see what flight I can catch."

Stella had no other comment or question; not about the funeral arrangements or the will, or how the house they had both been born in and in which Diane died would be disposed of; not one word in the year Stella was still reading newspapers and books, or in the years since.

My sister Eve was her closest friend. When Eve died of cancer Stella acknowledged the information as she had for Diane, and there was never another word, never a recollection, never an inquiry about Eve's children, or about her grandchildren who now had lost a whole set of grandparents to whom we were the successors.

Of all the peculiarities of Alzheimer's, the loss of empathy is to me the hardest to understand, and the first evidence of it came early, shortly before Loughrand's diagnosis. Stella said she was going to make an appointment to get her hair cut at the new beauty shop in the post office building. I thought I had missed something. I have a second-class memory and third-class hearing. Saying she was switching from Arlene's shop where she had had a regular appointment for twenty years was like saying out of the blue she would drop Grita. It wasn't something she would do because she got a coupon in the mail. Arlene was like family. Coupon bribery would be irrelevant, unheard of, impossible, and laughable. Her patronage would survive even a few bad haircuts and there hadn't been one. Arlene was good at what she did, knew her clients well, had unlimited tact and patience, and sane opinions on any topic in the news. She told fortunes, which were said to be astonishingly reliable, from soap suds. I thought she always got the cut right for Stella. I never heard Stella say otherwise.

I too had become a client of Arlene's after Stella said many husbands went to her and I braced myself to get my hair cut at something called a "beauty salon." For Stella to say without provocation that she was leaving Arlene for somebody she didn't even know — or leaving her for any reason — was beyond understanding. I blurted that she couldn't do that. What had brought it on?

"I've just decided, that's all."

"What am I supposed to tell Arlene when she asks about you?"

She shrugged.

"Just don't do anything like that until you think it over a long time. And then don't do it."

No cooperation was available from me. I had never before taken the part of any person in opposition to Stella. I took the other side on matters political or aesthetic, never in personal relationships. Her judgment about people was reliable and good enough for me.

The beauty shop in the post office building was not mentioned again.

Arlene's shop is a few steps up from street level. When Stella could no longer handle stairs Arlene began bringing her kit to the house. Today, Stella welcomes the news that Arlene is coming and enjoys the hour. When it is over, it is over. Unless Arlene reads this, she will never know that five years ago Stella might not have made the next appointment.

Why would Stella break so abruptly without reason or notice with a person who had been a true friend for twenty years? I can't explain it anymore than I can explain why she was so unmoved by the death of her sister and mine. I can't explain why she so enjoys the presence of her children and their families but never asks about them in their absence. She pays no attention when I talk to them on the phone or asks me questions when I hang up. If I hand her the phone, her face glows for the moments she hears their voices, as if hearing the first message on Alexander Graham Bell's new invention. She knows well who they are. She will say a yes or two. I take back the phone and she shows no more interest.

After I withdrew her from CenterDay, she did not once refer to it. After we had to give up BayEdge, not a word. No regret, no bewilderment, no loss. For two years, every day had been "Good day" at one of those day cares. The staffs had been like family. Never a word of memory.

I can't explain it, but knowing it I see its implications. Stella won't feel it very deeply or long if any or all of us — I, family, Grita — disappear from her life. She might miss Grita and me a little more and a little longer, but only a little.

Merck takes an oblique look at this: "All that [is] endearing to spouses, family, and friends is lost as the patient's mind, capabilities, sensitivities, and humanity disintegrate. Therefore, the appreciation that normally would be shown the caregiver of an elderly mate, parent, or friend is often missing."

To put it bleakly, if I step off a curb without looking both ways Stella will not long miss me. We have tested that. For two weeks, Grita went to Brazil to visit her parents. Stella may have had for moments a sense that something was missing but she never said it or showed it. I took a week to visit family and friends in distant states who were not as mobile as I. We did our best to have Stella understand that my absence was temporary, I would be back at the end of the week, although we knew that assurances embracing the passage of time were not functional for her. I telephoned every evening and spoke to her and Grita. Not until the third day did Stella acknowledge my absence to Grita.

"We were having lunch. She looked up and said, 'Where's Aaron?'"

"That's it?"

"I said you had to go away and would be back soon. She didn't say anymore about it."

Nor did she again. I was as relieved as I was disappointed. If I am absent from her life, she will not so much accept it as not notice it. Acceptance is deliberate, with a rankling undercurrent of regret. It can't be said that not taking notice has the same emotional force as accepting.

And yet, when she says, "Love you, dear," as she says one way or another every day without it staling — words, a glance, a hand held — it is not pro forma. It is not calculated — she has no calculation in her — the moment is transcendent.

But that card too will go back in her deck. Not much significance should be given if it is played once or twice in my absence. A third play is unlikely.

My intent to outlive her is not because losing me would be disorienting for her. I want to be here simply because I can do more for her than anybody else, even though she might not feel very profoundly or for very long the loss of whatever that is.

WILLISTON, another of my transient intimates in a caregiver group, said that when he had signed his wife into a nursing home, he thought it best not to come back too soon. He thought it would be like leaving a child at camp. If she was going to be homesick it would be early in the game; it would be better not to be around to be a crutch for her, it would only delay the adjustment; the staff was experienced with such situations and knew how to make the new resident feel at home.

He visited the nursing home a week later and spoke first to the staff person who said Mary was doing all right and soon would be well adjusted.

So she was not yet adjusted. He went to her room. She was sitting on a chair, looking out a window. Her greeting to him was beseeching. "I want to go home."

Williston said what Ina said, "It tears you up to hear something like that."

He did not take her home. It had been impossible before and would be impossible again. He had done his best and was still doing his best. If it was not this well-appointed, well-run nursing home it would be another no better.

How did he get away? How did he leave it with her?

"I wasn't great. I just kept snowing explanations on her and closing my ears. I told her she had to give it time. I said I would come often and her sister would come, that it was a fine place, she should think positively. She didn't hear any of it. When they came to toilet her and wash her up for dinner I got away. I asked them if she was like that when I was not there. Did she cry? The supervisor of the Alzheimer's unit said yes but that I shouldn't let it get to me. She was into their group activities. Give it time.

He gave it time. Once Williston's wife met him with a paper bag in hand she imagined to be packed for travel, and always, "'I want to go home.' I hated to go there and hear that and

I didn't know what to do about it. Then the focus changed, which made a big difference. Instead of talking about home she began to complain: the food had no flavor, it had too much salt, the laundry, the nurses, the podiatrist who came to cut her nails, the hair cutter, her clothes were being stolen. These were her reasons, justified or not, and I could deal with reasons.

"I assured her I would see what could be done. I talked to people. She was on a salt-free diet. They said they would have the table aide do something about condiments. Clothes were a little problem. There's a patient's rights thing that makes it unlawful to lock a resident's closet. The resident has to have free access. If the patient has free access, so does anybody else. I figured that staff helped themselves. They saw a raincoat they liked, the resident never went out in the rain, they took the coat. The floor supervisor said there might be some of that, but mostly things were lost, or the things had never existed, or residents took from residents. They had a man with a shoe fixation. Nothing they could do stopped him from dipping into somebody's closet and taking shoes."

I said to Williston that I guessed he could live with that.

"Anything is better than 'I want to go home.' You feel like a criminal. Do you want your wife to think you've done something awful to her?"

IT may be months or more before we miss them at the post office, the newsstand, the coffee shop, church. We see their wives or husbands alone where we would have expected them to be together. We haven't seen an obituary. We aren't family or close friends, but we know them. This is a small town; in a city it would be a neighborhood. This isn't a country where you're afraid to ask because the police may have taken him away.

"I haven't seen Wally Markle lately? Is he around?"

"Wally is in a nursing home."

A nursing home was never on my screen. My mother wasn't in a nursing home. My father at ninety-eight, a widower, full of disabilities, wasn't in a nursing home. When people asked, "Is Stella at home?" my inclination was to answer yes, implying forever.

Hearing that Stella, in an advanced stage of Alzheimer's, is at home, it is easy to assume that I share the widespread bias against nursing homes. I don't. If the time comes to sign myself in and I recognize it, I will do it with equanimity.

SOME years ago our good friend Fred Woodson, a bear of a man, was invaded by Alzheimer's. Esther, not half his size, coped for a long time, assisted by home-care aides, until it became too much for her. She signed Fred into a nursing home. At the same time, although still in good mental and physical health, she signed herself into the same twin-bedded room with adjoining sitting room and kitchenette. The facility's dining, housekeeping and health supports were available for their needs. It was very much like what came to be called assisted living.

They lived that way for several years until Fred died. By then it had become Esther's accustomed home. She died there uneventfully, physically frail but still knowing well her own mind. We visited Fred and Esther often. I thought Esther had made good choices.

If next Christmas marks the year Stella goes to a nursing home, I think about going with her, to keep an eye on her for as long as we have left. I wouldn't mind that at all. I have said to our children that I see no reason why their mother will not spend the rest of her life with me at home. I would not without their consent use my power as her husband or the durable power of attorney she signed to me (we to each other, then) six years ago to place her in a nursing home.

But I have also said that, should I in their judgment lose the power of reasonable decision for myself, no imagined prejudice or reluctance of mine should make their decision difficult. They should go ahead and sign me in. I have no reservation. I don't fear my children. I am lucky enough to have unlimited faith in them. What would displease me would be their not doing what seemed best because they supposed I would not want it if it were still my decision to make. If I have to be fed, the aides in a nursing home may feed me a little more hurriedly, there may be more soft foods to make meals go quickly and fewer playful foods like an apricot after dessert. My children may suspect that I will notice that people around me are sleeping in wheelchairs (as I may be) and that in some ways I may see it as a depreciated environment that will lessen my will to live. All this may be true, but my sense is that it will not matter greatly to me.

I don't begin with a prejudice against nursing homes for myself or Stella. For now, as far as I can see, our home is better. That's why we're here.

CAREER is a word we associate with employment at one's best skill. If the commitment isn't full time or intended to be, it is thought of as a hobby, but hobby is an insufficiently serious word for Stella's skill and her attachment to her cello. It seems to me that it happens less of a musician than of a painter, and certainly of a writer, that others think there must be something unfulfilled in the accomplished amateur who does not make a living, or at least suffer reputable starvation, at a professional level. Certainly it was not true of Stella. She was very good at what she did, she simply was not attracted to a career in performance. She played with several excellent string groups whose other members often had professional employment. She led the cello section of the county orchestra. She practiced strictly and daily. Her performance of the Bach suites for unaccompanied cello was reviewed as a fully professional performance by competent critics.

In a brief few months, her plan to gather a company of cellists to perform Villa-Lobos's "Bachianas Brasileiro #9" was wrecked by Alzheimer's. I saw calamity approach in her increasing inability to practice, to concentrate, to bring loose ends together, to remember where she put memos of telephone conversations.

At times I thought she was tired. At other times the pressure seemed to be getting to her. Her ordinarily level temperament seemed to be under compression. When the cello project began, her Alzheimer's had not yet been diagnosed. With the diagnosis came the realization that I had to in some way rescue her from an obligation with extensive responsibilities to a lot of people.

I called her local colleagues whom I, the dutiful spouse, knew from musical occasions. Simon Walsterman and Emma Blake had been to our house and we had been to theirs to unwind after performances. I think they were members of our church; at least they attended as much as we did. They were shocked and sympathetic and said they wanted to go on with the project. I did not propose managerial responsibility and they did not volunteer. They asked if I had spoken to Ben Casselli. I had not but I intended to.

Not wanting word-of-mouth to get too far ahead of me, on the same Sunday afternoon I visited Suzanna Kelley whom I had also met over wine and cheese and saw at the post office. Suzanna was a friend of Stella's and had a busy life as teacher and husbandless mother. She had visited us Christmas day with her preschool-age daughter. There had been an exchange of gifts — a bow-tied candy cane for a bracelet charm. Suzanna was also dismayed and asked if I had talked to Ben Castelli, so I understood that Castelli was somebody the ensemble would be comfortable with.

I remembered him as a tall man with bristly red hair drawn into a ponytail at one end and a Hapsburg beard on the other and a general air of emaciation as if from a diet of grassy health food. He lived at the end of the Cape. I telephoned and said bluntly that Stella was ill and I wanted to sit down with him before saying anymore.

"Oh dear," he said, "that doesn't sound very promising."

Neither did he, but he was all I knew to work with.

"You don't have to come all the way down here to talk," he said.

I said I would rather see him and could be there in an hour if he could see me. He gave me directions and within the hour I arrived at an imposing residence with a large entrance hall and a stairway of auditorium dimensions leading to a second-floor balcony. It was a purposeful house the owner had imagined in every detail and seen through to the end. We sat in a room of white wicker and plants. I didn't know firmly what I was going to propose.

"Oh dear, I am so sorry to hear this. Stell is such a nice person. Will she be able to play if the dog work is picked up by somebody else?" I was beginning to feel a rapport with him. He wasn't distancing himself.

"I can't be sure. The honest answer is I don't know. She is deeply committed. I'm sure the rest of you are too. It would be very hurtful to Stella if it were abandoned. The first question is, will somebody else do what you call the dog work."

"Excuse me," he said to pick up a ringing phone.

"Yes," he said, "Aaron is here now. We're talking. You want to stay with it, don't you? Of course. I'll call you back." So it was done.

"What about Stell?" he asked. "Can you take her through the adjustments all right? Would she accept that all right?"

I thought I could find the moments and the language to make it happen in an easy way. I said, "We've been married a long time. I think I know my way around."

"Oh dear," he said. "Life can be such a task. Call me when I can come to see you both and Stell can bring me up to date. Give her my love. She is such a nice person."

On an evening during the spring school break, our cavalcade of family cars — down from New York, up from Washington, my sister's son and family from Philadelphia — children, spouses, grandchildren, and Grita pulled into the parking lot of the high school at the stage door. Quite a few people were in their seats when we came into the aisle beside the stage and made our way to the rows that had been reserved. In a small town there are people to wave to, but Stella was entirely unselfconscious of it as an occasion in her life.

All sense of personal engagement with the concert had departed. Inch by inch, without visible regret, she had withdrawn from paperwork, from performance after a single short rehearsal, and then even from involvement of her emotions in the project she had so long anticipated. Eight cellos! had become just another evening out, the memorable part being her young family around her. The immediate and tiring pleasure of having all the children in the house at once had been enough for this day.

On stage, eight chairs were arranged in a shallow arc, each with a music stand and cello awaiting its artist. The houselights dimmed. Without announcement, three players took their places, acknowledged the welcoming applause, and bowed into a group of preliminary short pieces. After applause, for the set the other players came out briskly in black performance clothes. Two of the men were negligently put together, evidencing a conviction that a white shirt was the only essential. The women showed more the strain of being in costume. Margins of white shoulder strap slipped out. One had matched a flaring skirt to flaring hair for a pagoda-like effect. They had come to play. Slim and well tailored, Casselli stepped forward.

"You are here, I believe, for the 'Bachianas Brasileiro #9' by the Brazilian composer Heitor Villa-Lobos. I would like to say — and say now — that the performance was inspired and organized by our dear colleague Stella Alterra, to whom we dedicate the performance. Without her it would not have happened."

He extended his hand toward her and the audience accepted the invitation to applaud, rising in the ragged way audiences do when a few give the lead.

Stella did not get the full import of what Ben said. Her countenance was both serene and inattentive. I said to her, "The applause is for you. You have to show Ben your appreciation for his kind words. Throw him a kiss."

"A kiss?"

"Yes, throw him a kiss."

She did. Marion, sitting on my other side, leaned across and said, "That isn't all that wouldn't have happened without you, Mom."

Ben took his seat, the fine-tuning scraped to an end, he nodded the performance to begin, and at last Stella showed that she knew why she was there. She was there for the music, the wonderfully muscular, lyrical music. Her attention became intense. Her lips parted as if to drink in the voices of the cellos. Her attention did not waver until released by the closing applause and Ben Casselli motioning her to rise and accept it.

Ben came to visit her but not again and none of the others came ever. Friends — all but the treasured few — simply disappear into private discomfort, unease, embarrassment, distaste, fear, or other compelling interests. They cease to exist. That is as much the natural course of Alzheimer's disease as all that is written or implied in *The Merck Manual of Geriatrics.*

THE storm door has to be kicked to make a quarter circle in the snow at the front door. Lashed by the northeaster, the snow comes in flat out, wet; too much is down for the car to ram a lane from the garage to the neighborhood road. The stuff will pack, cement the car to the driveway, block the plow when it gets here. No newspapers! Snowed in. Power not gone, but soon. Even in mild storms I reset eight clocks and the VCR.

A March storm. In a week there will be nothing but shallow, dirty crusts to show for the mountains of snow at the edges of the parking lots and shoved in front of private driveways by the plows of higher authority.

The telephone works.

Marvin is out there somewhere shoving snow off town

roads or supermarket lots. I get him on his cell, remind him I have an invalid in the house. He thinks early afternoon. He won't be able to get in until the contractor does our road but he will keep his eye on it.

The fire department can probably get in if there is an emergency. Right now they aren't too concerned. The forecast is for less than eight inches, ending around noon. They are opening a shelter in the middle school just in case. Call them if I need them.

Shelley, the admissions officer at BayEdge Nursing and Convalescent, won't be at her desk yet. I leave a message reminding her that she agreed to take Mrs. Alterra for a day or a week in an emergency. Today or tomorrow might be the day. We would be all right here without heat for twenty-four hours but I wouldn't want to go beyond that.

It's Joan's duty day. Joan isn't looking for reasons to stay home. I suggest that she work her way down the highway to the Texaco and call me around noon. I will then know better if she can get in. "I can walk in from there," she says. Two miles.

Grita. My line has been busy. Her Wednesday client is in the hospital. If Joan doesn't get in, maybe she can. She lives closer. I thank her. If I need her I'll call. Stella has the two best aides on Cape Cod.

One more call. Emily Morse, a widow who lives alone farther down the road, will want somebody to tell her what's going on. I do that, as far as I know. She blesses me. She asks how Stella is. Fine. Sleeping.

I would just as soon that this be one of those mornings Stella wants to sleep until noon when Joan may have broken through, but she is stirring under the quilt, invisible, dug in as usual a half-dozen inches below the hemline. I drop a side rail, sit beside her, and peel my way in. Her eyes emerge aware that her cocoon is being unlayered. I kiss her and tell her how it is out there. I notice that the clock has stopped. I try a light switch. No power. Heat will soon begin to leak out of the house.

"Nobody here but us chickens," I tell her cheerfully. "Joan and Grita are snowed in too. Somebody will come in later. Right now it's just us chickens."

She reads me that I intend to be amusing. She smiles supportively.

I will leave the bathing to Joan and just get Stella out of her wet nightclothes, scrubbed with washcloths, dried, lotioned, powdered, and into a fresh gown. While I work I go on about whatever is relevant: the weather, the condition of her skin, her clothes. I get around to what a good sleeper she is.

"It must feel good to sleep all night."

"Good," she agrees, the first she has spoken, and closes her eyes. Who can blame her. The company is not scintillating. She is lying on her side, tucked into her fetal curl, clean and refreshed, ready for a nap.

I try again. "Why do you think you sleep so well these nights? You hardly move a finger. How do you account for that?"

She doesn't account.

"Do you remember what a restless sleeper you were?"

She doesn't remember, at least she doesn't admit it.

"When we were first married, you and I were holy rollers. Some nights I had all the blankets wound around me. Some nights you did. Do you remember that?"

She makes a noise I can't identify as a word. I take her hand and thumb it. Her fingers convulse around mine. Her eyes are closed.

I ask again how she accounts for her new gift of sleep and recall again for her how it used to be. Her voice stirs. I lean in to catch what she may say. I don't necessarily expect an answer and certainly not an elaborate one.

"It plays on a different reed," she says distinctly.

I don't know what it means but it is a lovely shard of poetry. Of all that we have said to each other in our long lives I think I will remember that sentence best.

I take her aloft in the Hoyer Lift and wheel her to a chair where she can watch snow come down. I think we have already lost a fraction of a degree of heat but it may be my imagination. "It plays on a different reed" keeps turning in my mind like a delightful toy that has a secret inside if I only knew how to get it open.

CODA

Here seems to be a good place to lead Stella the musician away and restore Virginia, the artist, to her rightful name and vocation. No events recounted in this memoir were more than mildly distorted, and those distortions were for the story to cohere. The characters, the conversations, and the events (except the orchestral interlude in the high school auditorium which really was an opening in the old town hall art gallery) were as a conscientious historian might reconstruct them.

Virginia, whose identity I chose to shield in her lifetime, should now be rightly identified as Virginia Brickley Harris, daughter of Clarence Mulford Harris, an ear, nose, and throat physician, and his wife, Bess Brickley. Their house in suburban Johnstown, Pennsylvania, was classic Midwest American, on a street with a grass strip down the middle and nearly a mile of elm trees, preserved from blight by the drip of fungicide in bottles strapped to their trunks. The house had a deep porch across the front, four bedrooms upstairs, and a bath. One bedroom was for Dr. and Bess Harris, one for Virginia, and another for her older sister, Betty. The fourth served as a sewing room and library. The suburb was Westmont, on a high hill above the gritty railroad city that drowned when the famous dam burst in the narrow valley.

Virginia's ancestry was Protestant, Scotch-Irish and perhaps Viking, while my forebears have been Jews forever. She had a long, narrow Yankee head and wore a size-ten dress for as long as I knew her. She earned her BA at Hood College, where she was in the dance club. She then took a graduate year at Simmons in Boston to study retailing and another year in apprentice training at Ivy's, a department store in Charlotte, North Carolina.

Bright, disciplined, and good-looking, Virginia had a choice of several permanent jobs in good stores. She accepted Kaufmann's in Pittsburgh, a major store whose peers between New York and Chicago—Wanamaker's in Philadelphia and Hudson's in Detroit—each offered her employment. But the Pittsburgh store was nearer her home and had exciting architectural renovations underway. Anything going on in art had her attention, then and for the rest of her life.

Kaufmann's was a big store with buying offices in New York and overseas. Its buyers had travel budgets to anywhere interesting articles might be found. The new young woman in the personnel department had many people to meet and much to learn. On her way through the store one day, she exchanged glances with a young man in the ad department. I have explained in earlier pages how I fell for her. Our marriage six months later endured for sixty-four years, until her death with Alzheimer's Disease at our home on Cape Cod in 2002.

Virginia became an accomplished artist. Painting, drawing, etching, creating collages, she welcomed new techniques. She was interested in people, nature, books, newspapers, the school life of our children, Richard and Susan. During her years as a sociology teacher at The Hartridge School, she thought up a course in, researched, and taught "Negro History" (long before it was conceivable to call it "Black History"). She picketed the Plainfield Country Club, protesting that citizens who were barred from membership by color or religion were obliged to meet there on public business. But she was, by nature, a peacemaker more than an activist, a community builder, and our family was her first community.

Alzheimer's is not a doctor's disease. It belongs to caregivers—family, nurses, aides—who see the patient through the long affliction for which there is no cure and no clear guidelines of what to expect at any stage. Virginia lost her ability to walk in the third year and lived seven years more in slow decline of strength and faculties. Many Alzheimer's patients, with more rapid and evident cognitive decline, never need a wheelchair at all. Doctors see Alzheimer's patients only occasionally. They look for treatable collateral problems, such as lung and kidney infections, that are seen in scans and blood tests and treated by prescriptions. They try new drugs, as they become available. Virginia's experience with Tacrine, the only Alzheimer's medication available in the early 1990s, had little effect except to upset her stomach. When Aricept (donepezil) became available, we switched. The new drug also had no useful effect but was easier on Virginia's digestion.

The first medication that seemed to have a positive impact on her Alzheimer's was Nemenda (memantine), a Swiss drug we heard about from friends in Florida. Alzheimer's had come to be understood as a siege inside the brain from several sources, and if more than one drug at a time were deployed, how could anyone know which drug worked? Namenda was the first drug joined with others to try for a synergistic or symbiotic effect. Virginia had an encouraging few weeks before Namenda, too, fell short of her need and she passed beyond the reach of medicine.

When Virginia was first diagnosed, in the early 1990s, my attention snagged on a number: there were four and a half million Alzheimer's cases in the United States. In the next decade, Alzheimer's became one of the darlings of medical journalism, with stories appearing about the vulnerable aging population, nursing homes, and research projects. The number of diagnosed cases swelled to 4,800,000 by 2002. All that investment, that promising research, that good news, and there were more cases than when they began the count?

Of course. What had been senility was now Alzheimer's Disease. Cases were sought and found in back bedrooms, in unofficial home-cares, buried in the figures of other diseases. A lot of elderly pneumonia was first Alzheimer's. The wonder was not that there was much more Alzheimer's than there had been ten years before but, with so little medication being conclusively helpful, that there was not even more.

The growing number of Alzheimer's patients may be outside the immediate concerns of doctors, but they are very much on the agenda of caregivers. In Virginia's years with Alzheimer's, while her physical and mental well-being dissolved, she suffered no pain. There was discomfort, and there was bewilderment that so much going on around her with familiar and unfamiliar people seemed to be not quite real, as if she were in a movie.

Virginia did not have to deal with the obstacles and dilemmas that her illness presented. Whatever the situation happened to be—an arm for which there was no sleeve, a door sill blocking her wheelchair—she waited for others to notice she was stuck. I think she would have sat in the wheelchair all night, gradually drifting to sleep, without showing any sign of discomfort beyond mild restlessness. The gift of raising her voice to call for a hand was also taken away in an early year. The caregiver is the patient's mentor, her eyes, her voice, the experience she lives in.

Palliative care became my agenda, but it was not within my range of ready understanding. I understood treatment and cure. I had survived the succession of childhood diseases— mumps, measles, scarlet fever, and flu during the post-World War II epidemic. Although I welcomed everything hopeful, I did not quite understand—or admit I understood—that every Alzheimer's drug was expected to fail after a year or two and was deployed only to hold the fort until then.

I think I know the event that conditioned me toward optimism about medical outcomes. When I was eight years old, I had double mastoiditis, which my mother explained as a kind of bone-rot behind my ears. The area was near the brain, the prognosis poor, but the sainted Dr. Gross went in there with his tools, cleaned out the rot, and soon had me home, never again to endure as much as an earache. I can recall the smell of iodide and the rude, scraping noise made inside my head drum by gauze drain strips being withdrawn from the wounds. This memory is not forbidding; it is about getting better.

Today, mastoid infections almost never get as far as the operating table. A cut is made, penicillin is poured in, and the patient is sent home, instructed to return for a checkup the next week. That is what I understood to be the usual course of a disease once medical science took a good look at it. But Alzheimer's seemed to be an exception. Nobody had anything optimistic to say about Alzheimer's.

During her last two or three years, Virginia was seldom aware of the world around her. We were fortunate to be able to hire devoted, competent aides who were with her throughout the day. Usually she napped unless focused by an aide on some detail of eating or dressing that required her participation. She was taken from bed by a Hoyer Lift, a derrick-like device wheeled to her bedside, that lifted her on a canvas sheet so she could be transported in the manner of a picture-book stork delivering a baby, to the dining room or bathroom, essentially for a change of scenery. The Hoyer saved many stretches and lifts that might have led to disabling backaches—the occupational hazard of aides. The first few times the Hoyer carried Virginia aloft she seemed mildly apprehensive, but soon she rather enjoyed the flight.

Most nights, after an aide prepared Virginia for sleeping and lowered the light, I pulled up a chair beside her bed so we faced each other, and I held her hand and talked for as long as she stayed awake about people or events she might recall. Some nights she would be asleep in a few minutes, or it might be an hour. The conversation was not entirely one-sided; occasionally I was rewarded by a small sound or her hand squeezing, which I took to have more content or recognition than may really have been there. How could I think otherwise when I knew how much was stored, if lost, inside her?

Then came the night I knew it was all over for her. I was not a stranger to the last passage before death. I had sat beside my mother's bed, relieving my father's watch, during the hours she breathed life away at home in Pittsburgh. I had sat beside my sister at the hospital, wishing her son through flight schedules and airport delays to make it from California in time for a last good-bye. Sam Glueck, my old friend from Pittsburgh and Plainfield, had his new wife summon me to North Carolina on what he sensed was his last day. When I got there, he focused out of a dream long enough to say my name and reach a wavering hand, before resuming the odd restless motions called motoring. His head slowly turned side to side, his hands wandered over the blanket coverlet. And he began the huge effort to breathe, like a steam train in a station. It went on for hours for Sam, as it had for my mother and my sister, and as it did that night for Virginia.

I called our children around midnight to say that their mother's life was nearly over. The entire final act was as I had experienced with the others. She was comfortable and in no distress except for the enormous effort to get enough air, as if she had run a race a mile longer than any she had imagined herself capable of and now—from what unimaginable resource?—was running another and then another.

Dick would arrive from Newton in an hour or so. Susan had farther to come and would be in before dawn. The love they had for their mother was not pro forma. They were now parents themselves and knew well that the familiar word has a particular meaning, more than any other in the language, to those lucky enough to have experienced it as they had. They truly loved their mother and knew they had been loved.

I worked then from the master Zeno's checklist of small, necessary, infinitely divisible things to do: I called Maria, housekeeper, caregiver, friend for so many years, who is identified as "Grita" in early chapters of this book. I called the hospice nurse who had not only nursely but also legal duties: documents for the coroner and for the department of health.

And so she died. The funeral home had known for a month that it might be one day soon. I let them know this was the day, it was over, and drove over there to see to the final arrangements. Their people were already on the way to bring Virginia in for preparation and viewing. Virginia would rest in the simplest of caskets. There would be flowers. They gave me the name and address of the florist so I could monitor the selection.

I came again later in the day with the children to look for the last time at her fine high-bridged Yankee profile. They had prepared her well, although they would not know the trace of her sidelong smile making its way through a crowded room, asking, "Isn't it time to go?" I widened my eyes and signaled, "Yes" before I caught myself acting inappropriately and straightened my face. Tomorrow she would be transferred to the furnace building and reduced to ashes. Friday I would call for her remains.

The memorial service remained to be planned. It would not be a religious service with hymns and readings and prayers, which she specifically did not want, but rather a simple gathering of family and friends. I tried to think about it as Virginia would have. Because the omission of any religious statement might be troubling to many of those present, the Unitarian minister would lead off. We had been supportive members for decades of the church's institutional mission to be an open door to those of every faith or no faith at all who choose to come together. Then family members and a few dear friends would speak about Virginia. We would gather in our house and garden, weather permitting. If not, she would like the environment of the handsome new senior center where some of her paintings and the paintings of friends were hung.

The small metal box stayed on my desk for a month before there was a fresh and sunny morning that felt right to walk it down the path to the river and empty it on the out-tide, surprised that there was not only ash but fragments of charred bone. The tide eddied briefly before taking her into the current. I watched until the drift disappeared in my wet eyes.

ABOUT THE AUTHOR

"AARON ALTERRA" is a pen name for E. S. GOLDMAN, the author of numerous stories published in the *Atlantic Monthly* and other periodicals, two story collections, a novel, and a book of poetry. He resides on Cape Cod, in Massachusetts.